The Perks of Having Cancer

An Inspirational, Positive and Humorous View of a Not-So-Inspirational, Positive or Humorous Situation

By Diana Bosse, Cancer Survivor
Illustrated by Steve Wallace

THE PERKS OF HAVING CANCER

An Inspirational, Positive and Humorous View of a
Not-So-Inspirational, Positive or Humorous Situation

ISBN 978-1-7339955-1-1

For information, contact the author:

Diana Bosse
1721 Old Farm Dr.
Loveland, OH 45140
dianabosse@aol.com

Published by:

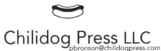

Chilidog Press LLC
pbronson@chilidogpress.com

Chilidog Press LLC
Loveland, Ohio
www.chilidogpress.com

Illustrated by Steve Wallace
Book Design by Andy Melchers

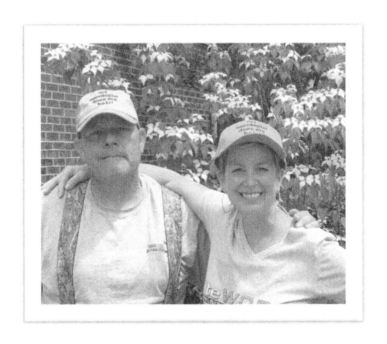

In Memory of Charlie

This book is dedicated to the many people who helped me laugh so I could live

My husband, Steve: My best friend, my primary caregiver, my rock, my love and the most important person in my life. ALWAYS.

In remembrance of my parents, Pat and Bill Cordry: Although they didn't give me life, they certainly taught me how to live.

Big Poppa: The man who gave me life and a warped sense of humor.

Dr. Chua and the staff at Oncology Hematology Care: You saved my life.

The HHIPS (Hilton Head Island Princess Society): My best friends for life – Tammy and Marianne (since 1962), Anne (1967), Shawna (1971), Gina and Barb (1976), Marlene (1983), Laura (1984), Sharyn (1993).

My Co-workers at the Alzheimer's Association of Greater Cincinnati: Their work-life balance was out of kilter already, but they did double duty covering me when I was on medical leave for nearly five months. I am forever grateful.

My friends from St. Columban Church: The foundation of my spiritual life.

My inspirations: Mark and Krista – Cancer survivors with a zest for life.

Relatives: My sister, Nancy, and especially cousin Diane who holds the family together and has ministered to the sick her entire life.

Friends: There are too many to mention, but am blessed to have each and every one of you in my life.

Folks from my past life that I reconnected with on Facebook: Including Kelly and Randy who were diagnosed with cancer about the same time as me. We rode the roller coaster together with minimal barfing.

People I barely know

And above all, God: With His love and the many "winks" He sent me, I was never afraid. EVER.

Table of Contents

PREFACE

It's only cancer. As blasé as that may sound, I work for the Alzheimer's Association. Alzheimer's disease has no effective treatment. No prevention. No cure. It's always fatal. So, when the doctor came into the emergency room at 3:30 a.m. on April 12, 2019 and said to me, "You do not have a bowel obstruction (good news?). The CAT scan shows extensive swelling in the lymph nodes of your abdomen which indicates cancer."

My first thought was, *"SERIOUSLY?"*

My second thought was, *"Maybe I should have told my husband to meet me at the ER."*

My third thought was, *"At least it isn't Alzheimer's. With cancer I have a chance."*

As I laid alone with my thoughts waiting for my husband to arrive and for a room to open on the oncology floor, I resolved to remain positive throughout this journey, thus improving my chances. Since humor is my default coping mechanism, laughing through lymphoma came naturally. I began posting daily "Perks of Having Cancer" on Facebook, making my business everyone else's business too. To my surprise, people were inspired and encouraged by my writing. In return, they inspired and encouraged me.

As the days and weeks of treatment passed, I realized "The Perks" might make a great book. I've always believed there is a purpose for everything. By sharing my own journey over the next six months, I could lift others in theirs. This was my purpose.

Plus, I have always wanted to be a published author.

And rich and famous.

One out of three ain't bad.

"A keen sense of humor helps us to overlook the unbecoming, understand the unconventional, tolerate the unpleasant, overcome the unexpected, and outlast the unbearable."

– Billy Graham

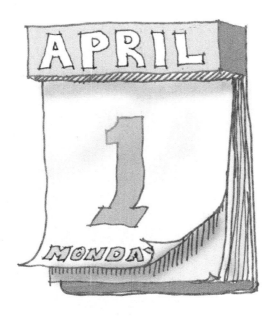

"If there's life, there is hope."

—Stephen Hawking

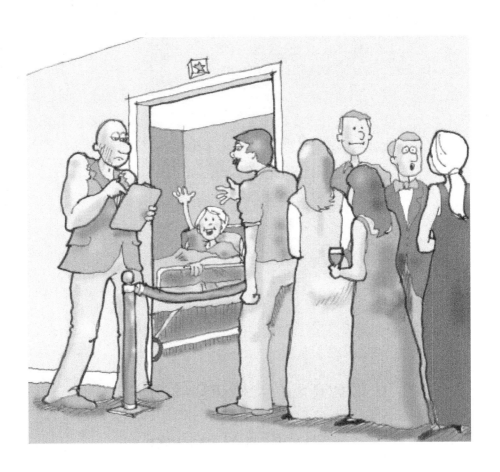

Star of Your Own Tear-Jerker Movie

People began arriving at the hospital early on Friday, April 12. At one point, the nurse said we were breaking all box office records by the number of fans lined up outside the door. Room 5221 was my theatre and the Hill-Rom hospital bed, my stage. Regardless of the shock from the diagnosis and subsequent turmoil in my head, I flashed a confident smile to everyone who came to see me. It was quite the performance... or maybe it was just the drugs. I felt like James Mason/Kris Kristofferson/Bradley Cooper in *A Star is Born*. I loved being the center of attention, despite not being a very good singer. I knew, however, that I was going to have to re-write the ending.

Thus, *The Perks of Having Cancer* was born.

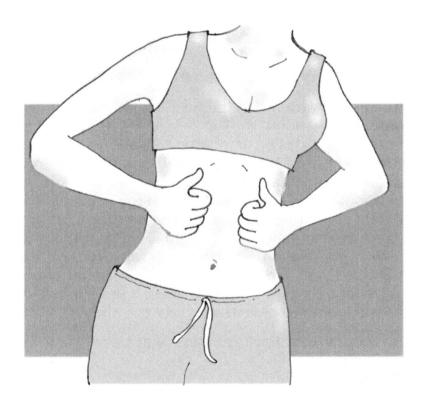

Great Abs at 56

Finding joy in cancer may not be easy, but it can have its perks. Chemo is covered by insurance. Cool Sculpting is not. Once all the swollen lymph nodes in my stomach are zapped, I expect to be bikini ready.

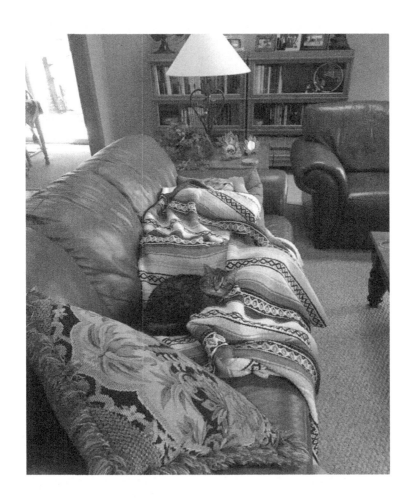

Laziness

You do not need to explain to anyone why you now sleep more than the cat.

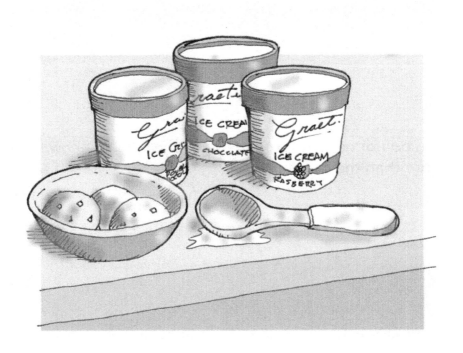

Getting Just About Anything You Want

Tell hubby you are craving ice cream and POOF... it magically appears! Tell hubby mac-and-cheese from a favorite BBQ joint sounds good and BAM... there it is! Tell hubby you'd like an ergonomic lounger to enjoy time outside on the patio and ZOOM... he's off to Bed, Bath & Beyond with coupons in hand! I wonder if I told him a twenty-eight-foot boat would cure me – would I finally get one? I already have the perfect name picked out – "The Boss Sea" (play on the ole' last name).

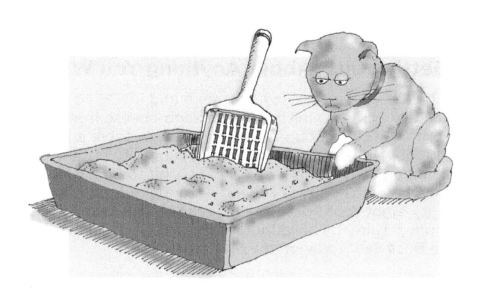

Dirty Jobs

I was crushed to learn that due to a weakened immune system, I could not clean our cat Maddy's litter box while going through treatment. As an added bonus, I was forbidden to wipe up any randomly hacked up hairballs. Therefore, when Steve comes home from a long day at work, I simply point (from my ergonomic lounger that is in the family room during inclement weather) to the "gift" on the carpet and he runs to find a rag and bottle of white vinegar.

I'm sure the same would apply to any dog owner.

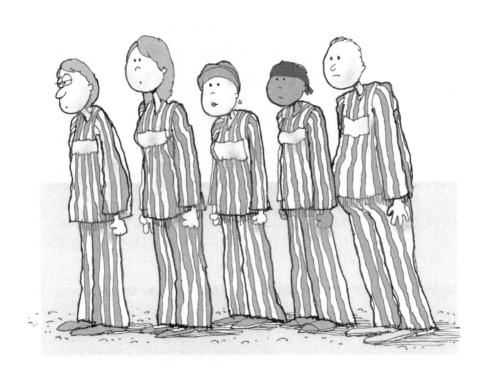

A New Identity

I am now Diana Bosse 09191962. Bosse has officially become my middle name and date of birth seemingly my last. Everyone at every appointment refers to you that way. Automatically add in the digits when the receptionist asks your name and you will impress them every time.

It sounds like I should be in prison.

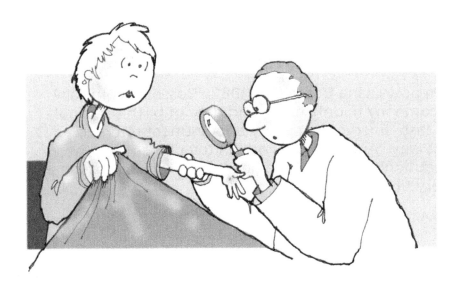

Port-o-Cath

I'm pretty sure every phlebotomist in the region is grateful I now have a port so they will no longer be perplexed as to how a living, breathing human being can survive without veins and blood.

I'm relieved I no longer have to be a human pin cushion. Plus, I have another reason to remind Steve that every "port" deserves a boat.

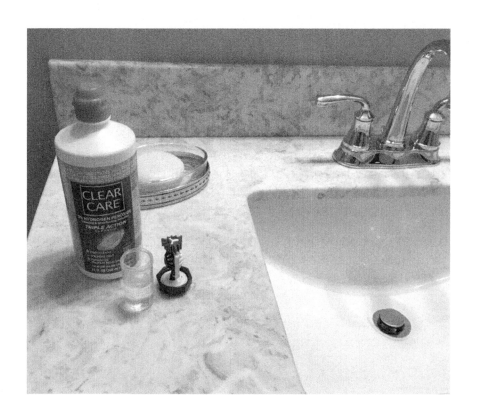

Chemo Brain

Trust me folks, you can blame every single stupid thing you do on "chemo brain." For example, I woke up one morning and sweet hubby asked if I needed anything. I said I wanted to relax in bed a bit longer, but could he bring me my phone? He did but I couldn't read a thing. I grabbed my readers from the nightstand and they helped, but my eyes were goopy and it seemed as if I was looking through a dense fog. I limped over a few messages and decided to get my bifocals. I put them on and it was worse—much worse.

Dear God, I was going blind. Not now! I have enough to deal with. Seriously?!? I don't recall any doctor or nurse telling me blindness was a side effect of treatment. Not one.

I dejectedly walked into the bathroom to pee for the sixty-seventh time since they pumped me full of a liter of meds and I drank what seemed like three of the five Great Lakes. That's when I saw my empty lens case and nighttime solution on the counter. I wasn't going blind. I slept in my contacts! I hadn't done that since my early twenties after a bottle of Peppermint Schnapps. Sleeping in your contacts really makes your eyes foggy and goopy and if you put other glasses on top, you have horrible vision.

Anywho, I'm relieved I'm not blind... just dumb. Thank you, chemo brain!

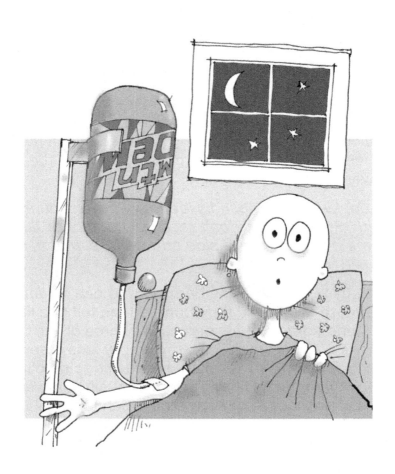

Insomnia

One of the side effects of prednisone is difficulty sleeping. My chemo cocktail happens to include prednisone. Plus, after each treatment I take five extra pills a day for five days. This is the equivalent to giving a two-liter of Mountain Dew intravenously to an insomniac. Now I just don't sleep at all. This, however, can come in very handy because I have a lot to do. It's currently 3:37 a.m. and I've written four thank-you notes and folded three loads of laundry. You can get stuff done, my friends!

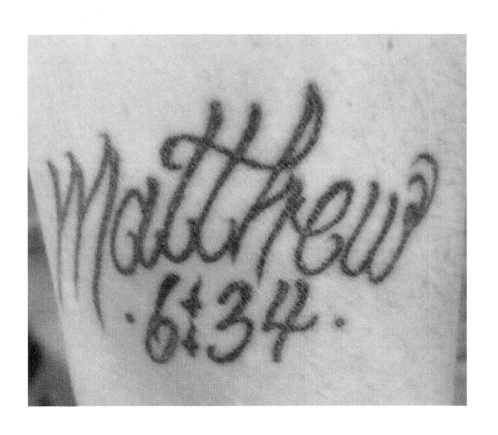

Worrying

If you like to worry, cancer is your disease! When you are first diagnosed, the unknowns are far greater than the knowns. I didn't know what lie ahead, so I did what I do best—I worried. I come from a long line of worriers—Mom and Grandma took the craft to a new level; therefore, I had no choice but to carry on the tradition. It doesn't help that I'm "allergic" to pain and vomiting and people are more than willing to share horror stories. IGNORE THEM.

Nothing so far has been as bad as I thought it would be or even anything more than uncomfortable. *Not even the bone marrow biopsy.* Heck, the anesthesiologist put me so far out, the doctor could have amputated my legs that day and I wouldn't have felt it or even cared. So, when some man (it's always the men that tell you how bad it was) tells you a procedure is so awful you will want to die, take it with a grain of salt—preferably around the rim of a margarita if your oncologist still allows you a cocktail every now and then.

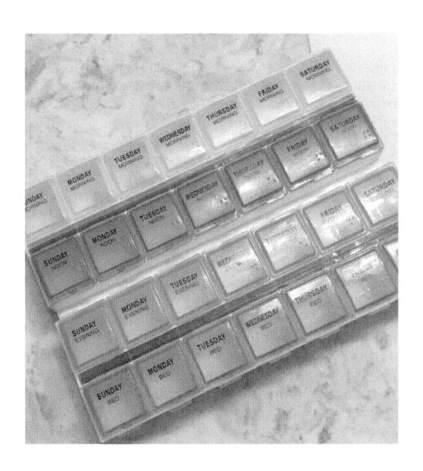

New Organizational Tools

I currently do laps at the pharmacy drive-through window. I have more pills than I know what to do with. I was excited when Steve found a pretty new multi-colored pillbox to get myself organized. I thought you had to be 65 or over for one of these gadgets. Or at least be a card-carrying AARP member. Apparently not!

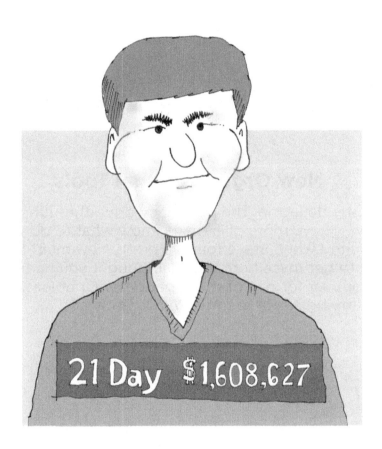

You Learn a Lot

I assimilated more medical terminology in three weeks than I did in all my science and biology classes combined. I can even spell lymphoma and several anti-nausea medications without the help of spellcheck. I may not be able to beat James Holzhauer on *Jeopardy!*, but if the Big C comes up when I'm on the show, I can pretty much run the category. That is, as long as chemo brain doesn't show up during the taping.

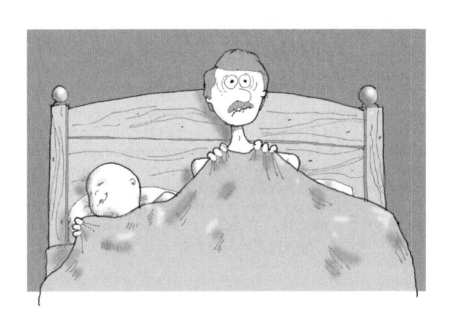

Not Tonight, Honey, I Had Chemo

Ladies, you will have a new excuse not to have sex!

As a part of our initial consultation prior to my first chemo treatment, the nurse had to have "the talk" with me and Steve. Apparently, this life-saving poison being injected into my body could be detrimental to my husband. In addition to flushing the toilet twice, if Steve and I should wish to make love, he needs to wear a condom. Since he's not carried one in his wallet since his college days, and a trip to the drug store seems like too much trouble, I can rest easy. That is, if only the prednisone would allow me to sleep...

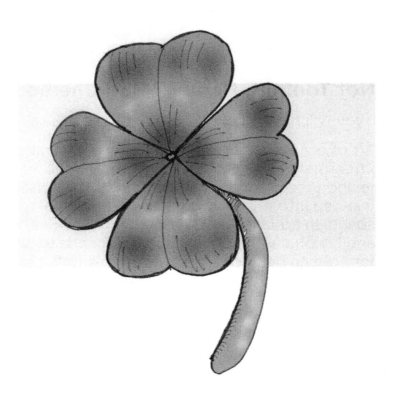

It's Like Christmas

You will receive greeting cards. Dozens of them. Flowers and fruit baskets arrive. An occasional gift is left on your doorstep from Amazon, UPS or Fed Ex. Sometimes... the best times... gifts are even dropped off in person by relatives and friends. People stop by.

One afternoon my birth father, aka Big Poppa, came with lunch, and later in the day Marianne popped in for a visit. Marianne has been a friend since I was born. She *is* my childhood. We chatted for hours, watched *Ellen* together, and when the skies cleared, we decided to take a walk around the short block. As we traversed the street, she commented on how we used to jump in puddles along the curb. We passed a yard that had a plethora of clover. We reminisced about making clover chain necklaces and sang "I'm Looking Over A Four-Leaf Clover," when I mentioned that I'd never found one before. I've looked for years, but the four-leaf variety have always eluded me. Marianne started searching at the edge of the lawn and within two minutes handed me the most perfect gift. She had never found a four-leaf clover either but insisted I take it. She must have known that with a lot of faith, good friends and a little luck, I can beat this thing. How lucky am I?

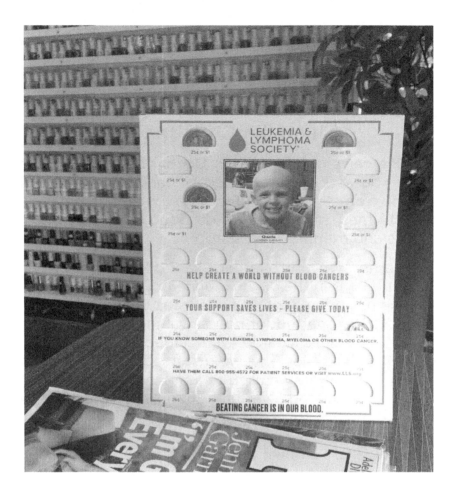

God Winks

Many people are spiritual or believe in something. I hope you have some type of faith to carry you through this thing called life. It can come in very handy during trying times. I happen to believe in God... and Jesus... and signs from both.

Early on in my journey, my dear friend Diana picked me up and took me to get a "mani-pedi." I actually have two dear friends named Diana and both their last names start with the letter B. What are the chances? The other Diana taught me about God Winks—a coincidence so astonishing that it is seen as a sign of divine intervention, especially when perceived as the answer to a prayer.

A God Wink is the basis of this perk.

The spa nail treatment was far more relaxing than any of the chemo treatments I was receiving at the time. At the end of the appointment, I joined Diana as she perched herself under the dryer. As I sat down, I noticed an old-fashioned cardboard coin cutout used to collect charitable donations. I saw the droplet of red blood first and knew immediately it was for the Leukemia and Lymphoma Society. I spied the photo of a perfectly bald head and thought "that will be me soon," but then noticed the incredible smile and the word in bold print beneath his name: SURVIVOR. I felt as if I was looking into a mirror, not a piece of cardboard. It was the God Wink I needed in that moment. The good Lord really "nailed" it.

Now Jesus did many other signs in the presence of his disciples that are not written in this book. But these are written that you may come to believe that Jesus is the Messiah, the Son of God and that through this belief you may have life in his name.

— John 20:30-31

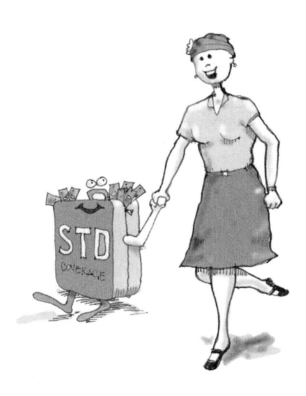

STD

Get your mind out of the gutter, please. It's not what you think. STD also stands for Short Term Disability. If you have a job that offers it, take advantage. Cancer will keep you busy between tests, procedures, infusions, calling insurance companies, writing thank you notes, sleeping... or not... meditating, feeling grateful to be alive, whatever. Your day will be jam-packed. Fill out the paperwork and get busy not working!

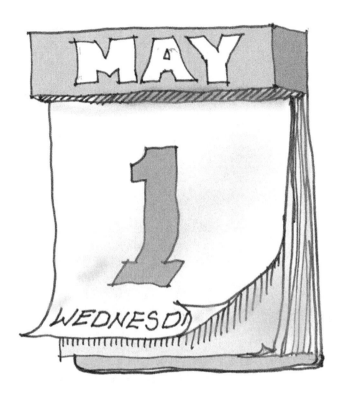

"First do what is necessary,

Then do what is possible,

and before long you will find
yourself doing the impossible."

—St. Francis of Assisi

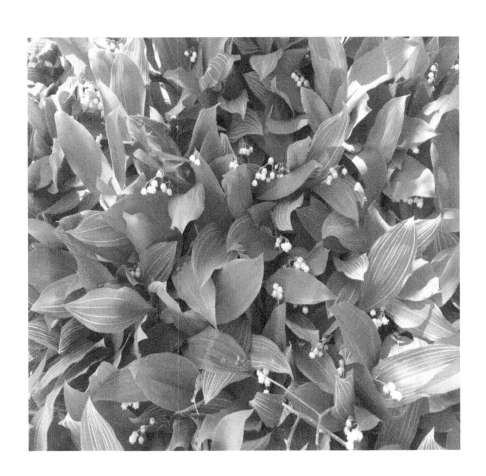

Stop and Smell the Roses
(or Whatever is Blooming)

Years ago, when Dad was sick and living with us, his illness taught me to slow down and appreciate nature, if only for a moment. Since his passing in 2008, life sped up again until cancer forced me off the merry-go-round.

One day as I walked in the neighborhood, I not only stopped, I practically laid down in a bed of lily-of-the-valley in my neighbors' front yard. I hope they were at work and didn't see me. If I knew for sure they *wouldn't* see me, I probably would have taken a trowel and dug up a few bulbs for Steve to plant in my own backyard. The fragrance was amazing!

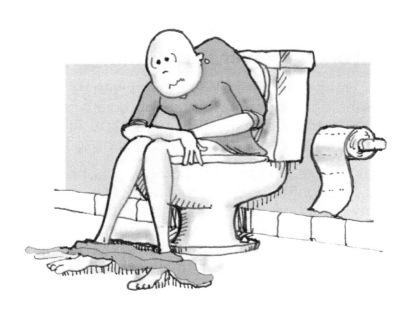

Toilet Paper

You will not blow your budget on double rolls of Quilted Northern Ultra Plus, as all the money spent on trips to the bathroom to pee will be offset by the lack of visits to do #2. Chemo binds you up! I haven't crapped since there was snow on the ground and it's now spring. There's a buzz of activity in my abdomen between the chemo kicking cancer's butt and this big hunk of poop navigating a leisurely cruise through my colon. I can literally feel it at every turn in my intestine like a baby kicking. I'm thinking about hiring a midwife for its arrival. Plus, Steve and I are having fun picking out names. We are leaning toward "Enema" if it's a girl.

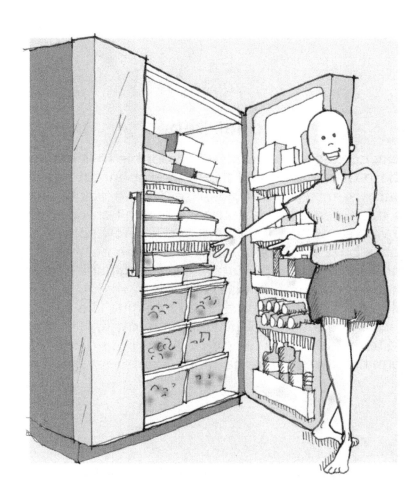

The Meal Train

I am fortunate to know a lot of people who also happen to be very good cooks. Not only did my friends sign me up for a prayer chain to feed my soul, they also signed me up for a meal train to feed the rest of me and Steve too! Several days a week a Good Samaritan magically appears at my front door with a delicious home-cooked meal that typically lasts a couple of days or can be frozen. It's coordinated so I don't get fourteen pans of lasagna, and thoughtfully prepared with Steve's low-sodium diet taken into consideration (he had congestive heart failure in the fall—it's been a helluva year). So even on the days when I don't feel like eating, he still gets to. Plus, my kitchen stays pristine. All aboard!

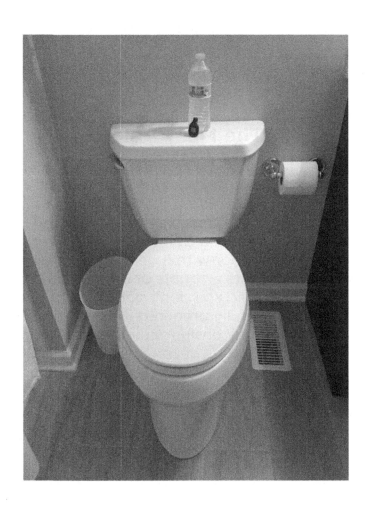

Complimentary Fitness Membership

Dad used to call water the "Elixir of Life." Water will be your best friend... and your worst. It is imperative to stay hydrated while going through chemo, which means you must drink the equivalent of Lake Erie each day. You will get all 10,000 Fitbit steps in as you slosh your way between the recliner and bathroom. To add upper body strength to your workout, use your right arm on the first flush and left on the second (with chemo, you must flush twice). It's quite the exercise program. No special equipment required!

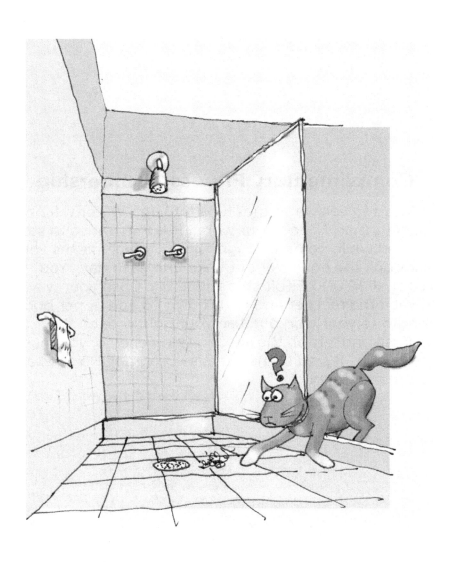

Blame the Hairballs on the Cat

As you discover an increasing amount of hair on your pillow, the bedroom carpet and the bathroom floor, you can convince yourself that it's just the cat. That is until you find the hairballs in the shower. Everyone knows cats hate water. Oh well, at least the chemo is doing its job!

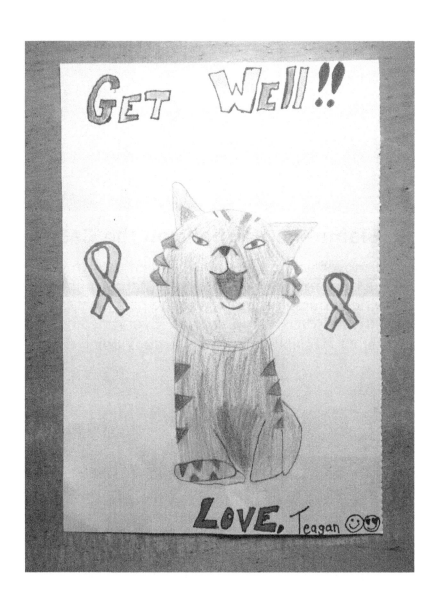

Artwork

You'll begin to accumulate priceless works of art. Who needs Monet or Renoir when you can have a beautiful drawing from your grandniece?

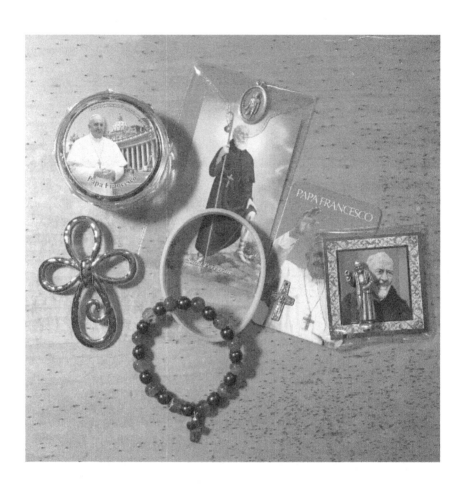

Jewelry

People will bequeath gifts far more valuable than gold, silver or even diamonds. Charms packaged with prayers from saints. Beads from holy churches in Europe, blessed by a priest. Colorful rubber bracelets for you, your husband and all your friends to wear to show their support. It's quite humbling.

With all these meaningful trinkets, you have no choice but to be healed and no chance that the devil will possess your body. EVER.

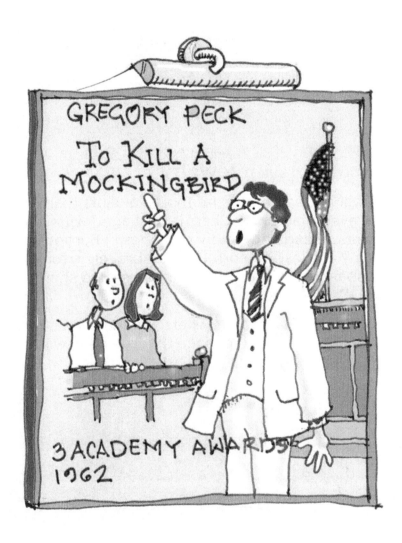

Classic Movies

Old friends will bring you old movies to help pass the time. Your oldest friends will come over to watch them with you. One rainy afternoon, Tammy and I watched To *Kill A Mockingbird*. Neither of us had ever seen it or even read the book. It was released the same year we were born and the same year we became the best of friends—1962. Now we know what all of the hype was about. It is fantastic.

"Scout" reminded me a bit of Tammy. Except Tammy was not a tomboy—on the contrary! She loved pink and owned six Polly Flinders dresses. But she did like to beat me up. One time I ran home crying, complaining to my parents that Tammy had hit me. Dad told me to go hit her back. I came home a little later, crying even harder. Dad asked what happened and I told him she wouldn't let me.

Today I am grateful to Tammy for toughening me up. With cancer, you need to be a fighter. Thanks to her love, support and a few right hooks over the last 56 years, I know I'm up for the battle.

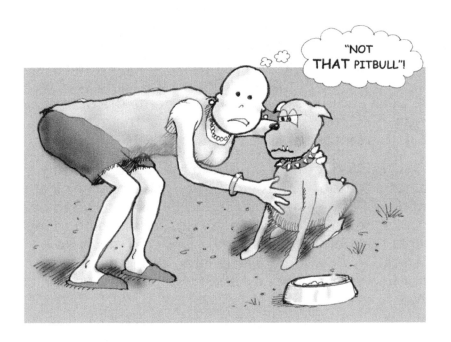

Gaining Celebrity Status

One day along your journey, you may find yourself mistaken for a celebrity. Sadly, in my case, it's the singer, rapper, songwriter and record producer Pitbull. Why does bald look so sexy on men? Me, not so much. I knew the day would come and it bothered me more than I thought it would, but I can still find positivity in losing my hair:

- I will gain back at least 15 minutes a day between washing, drying and styling.

- I'll save an additional hour a month for cut and color.

- Then there's the monetary benefits—no more shampoo, mousse, hairspray, electricity from the blow dryer and the cost of gas to get across town to see my stylist who kindly undercharged me to cut or color my hair (I hope she doesn't read this and raise her prices by the time my hair grows back).

- No more bad hair days.

- Free wigs.

- New hashtag #Mrs305

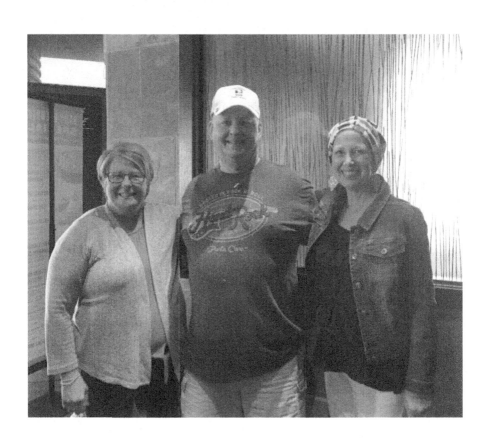

The Cancer Alumni Club

You can join support groups or clubs. You may even start one of your own, like I did. I had not seen Kelly and Randy in nearly forty years. As luck would have it, both were diagnosed around the same time I was. We were friends on Facebook and now have our own personal online support group via Messenger where we can compare fun stuff like who has the largest incision (Kelly) or discuss clogged ports (Randy) and lack of hair (yours truly). High school reunions are a great way to connect with old school chums, but a serious illness paired with Facebook works just as well. Plus, there is no special planning and you don't have to shop for the perfect outfit or worry if your significant other will be bored listening to previously untold stories about your old high-school sweetheart.

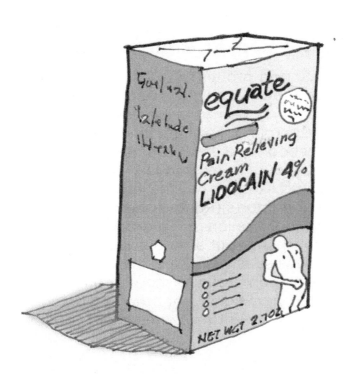

Numbing Cream

This is not a perk for me, but may be for others. I hear that if you use Lidocaine to numb the area around your port before they stick you with that very large needle, you don't feel a thing. Sadly, due to a certain type of medicine that is administered to me, I cannot be numbed prior to the gentle nurse pushing battery acid through my body. Apparently, if even a drop of the stuff escapes from my vein, it can cause extensive tissue damage and my left boob could potentially melt off right there in the recliner chair. I need to be able to feel if that is happening.

It's my assumption that the chemo drug Vincristine—despite its beautiful, melodious name—must be derived from some flesh-eating bacteria from somewhere in Africa. Nice!

Therefore, on my chemo visits, I'll deal with the pain. The good news is it's really not as bad as *that guy* told me it would be. The pain registers somewhere between a flu shot and a cortisone injection and the sting only lasts about ten seconds. Of course, you would not have guessed it by the lady sitting next to my husband during one of my treatments. When the nurse asked if she was ready, she clutched the arms of the recliner like she had just been buckled into a rollercoaster and immediately started Lamaze breathing techniques. I thought she was going to pass out. No, on second thought, maybe that was Steve...

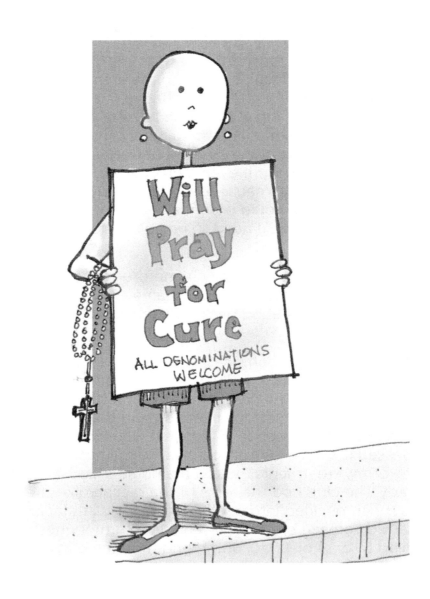

Access to the Most Powerful Drugs

I've been going to church every day like it's my job. I guess since I'm not working right now, it really *is* my job. That said, the reason I started doing so was two-fold:

1. I believe in the power of prayer; and,

2. It forced me to get out of bed every morning, take a shower and get dressed. Otherwise, I'd probably still be in my pajamas watching *Ellen* when Steve arrived home from work.

Communion is very important to me, and I have to admit I'm disappointed I cannot drink the wine as I'm going through treatment. Potential germs in the communal cup are probably a mortal sin. I considered asking Father Larry if I could bring my own flask, but thought he might frown upon that. The good news is I can still receive the host. The other day, as the wafer melted on my tongue, I realized the bread truly is the most powerful medication I'm currently receiving. It's Christ's "chemo." I KNOW I will be healed in Jesus's name. Amen!

"The bread that I will give, is my flesh for the life of the world, and if you eat of this bread, you shall live forever, you shall live forever. And I will raise you up, and I will raise you up, and I will raise you up on the last day."

– From the communion song,
"I Am the Bread of Life"

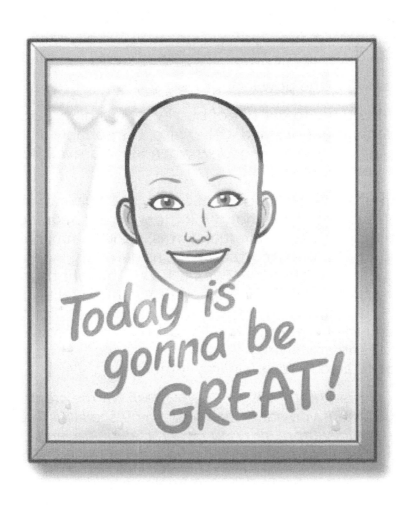

Bitmojis

You will have an excuse to update yours.

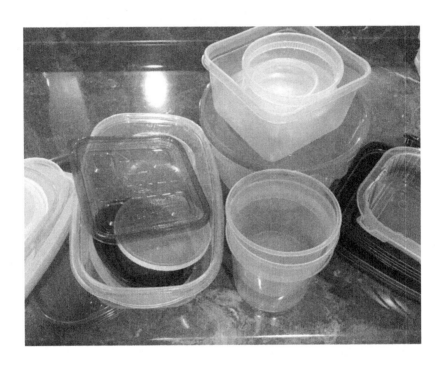

Plastic Food Containers

Once the tracks to the meal train are laid to your doorstep, an added benefit is that most food is delivered in nice, reusable containers. As people spread the buffet out on your spotless kitchen counter, they typically wave their hands and say, "Don't worry, I don't need anything back."

Jackpot!

Now my kitchen cabinets, linen closet, dry bar, bookshelves and half of Steve's basement workbench are stacked high with every imaginable size and shape of plastic ware. You must be careful, however, as there is a fine line between having enough and finding yourself on an episode of *Hoarding: Buried Alive*.

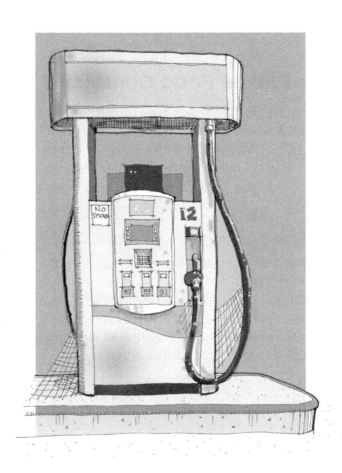

Driving

Apparently, when you have cancer your driver's license is automatically revoked. People insist on picking you up and driving you everywhere. Take advantage of this. I'm saving nearly $40 a week in medium grade unleaded.

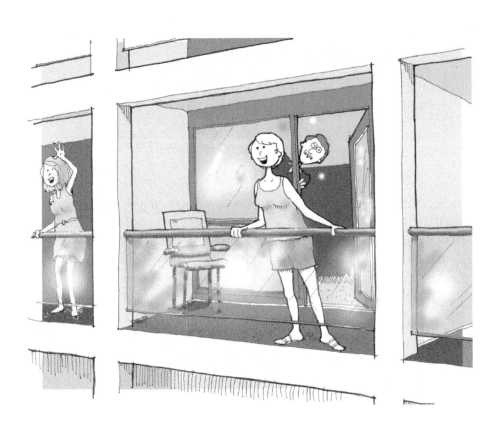

Come Sail Away

I love being on a boat—canoe, pontoon, motorboat, bass boat, yacht, cruise ship, kayak, raft. If it floats, I love it. Steve, not so much. Even if I won a gazillion dollars on *Jeopardy!*, he would never let me buy a boat. He's too practical. He says it's much smarter to rent one:

"Do you know how many times you can go deep sea fishing for four hours and you don't have to clean it, care for it or put gas in it and it only costs a couple hundred bucks?"

That's his argument. Therefore, I'll never truly *own* a boat. Unless I divorce him. But I love him, so that's not happening.

I also want to travel outside the United States again, but he does not.

"It's not safe!"

Safe? I work on Linn Street in the West End of Downtown Cincinnati. I'm more likely to get shot crossing the street to pick up a sandwich from Subway than I am to get killed in a terrorist attack. I'll take my chances in Paris, thank you!

That said, in my dire cancerous situation, Steve said to me, "When you get through all of this, I'll take you on a trip anywhere you want." Big mistake on his part because as soon as the words were out of his mouth, he knew it would involve a boat and a foreign country.

I've selected a lovely 8-day European Viking River Cruise. Bon Voyage!

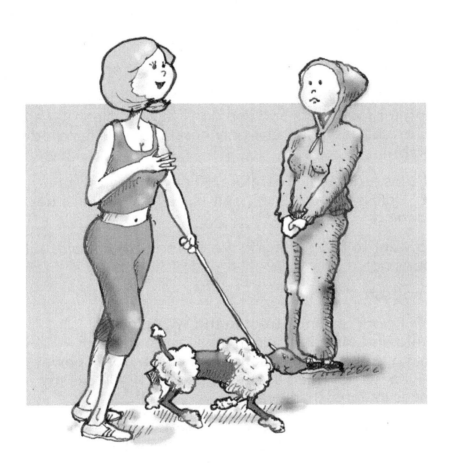

No Makeup

You have an excuse to look like hell and there will be days when you do not feel like doing anything to improve said looks. Of course, that will be the day you are on your morning walk and run into the perky neighbor with the cute hair style walking her dog with an equally attractive cut, and she says to you, "You look great!" She's just being polite because you know perfectly well you look like you were just liberated from Auschwitz with your gaunt cheeks, dark circles and bald head. Just bat your lash-less eyes, politely thank her, hold your shiny head high and move on.

And remember, at least you don't have to pick up dog poop!

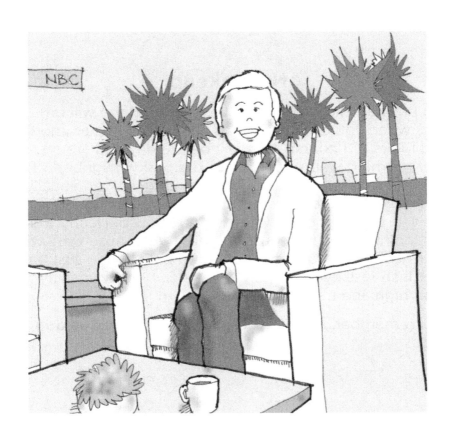

If You ARE a People Person, This is Your Disease

You will meet lots of people. They will want to know EVERYTHING about you. I watched the Ellen DeGeneres show the other day and she talked about people following her into the restroom to talk to her. I know the feeling. I hope to get on the *Ellen* show someday. I love her sense of humor and commitment to kindness. I think we'd have a lot to talk about outside of the restroom.

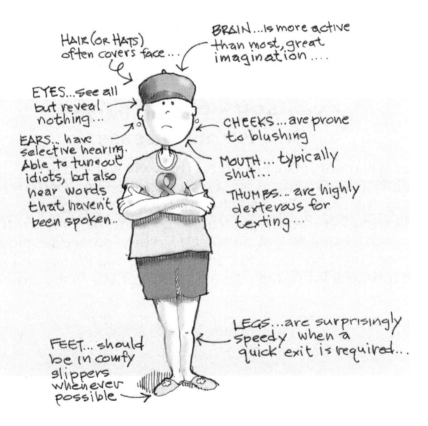

If You Are NOT a People Person, This is Your Disease

Along the journey, I've learned another new word—nadir. While it sounds like a picturesque city on a crystal-clear sea in the Mediterranean, nadir is defined in the dictionary as:

na·dir *noun*

1. the lowest point in the fortunes of a person or organization.
   "they had reached the nadir of their sufferings"

2. *synonyms:* the lowest point, the all-time low, the lowest level, low-water mark, the bottom, as low as one can get, rock-bottom, the depths; zero; *informal* "the pits."

Relative to chemo, it's the period in which your blood counts are the lowest. During nadir, it may be best to isolate yourself from others. This is great news if you are an introvert! This period typically falls seven days after chemo and lasts a good three to five days. Of course, you can always stretch it out and embellish your low blood count if you prefer more alone time. No one will ever know except your medical professionals.

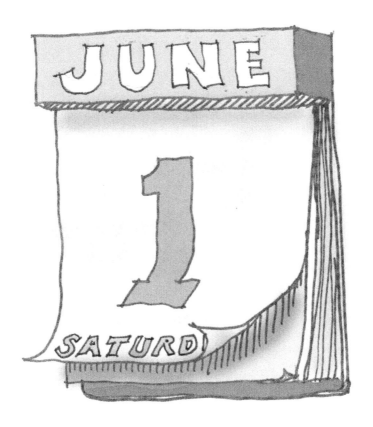

"Courage is resistance to fear, mastery of fear, not absence of fear."

—Mark Twain

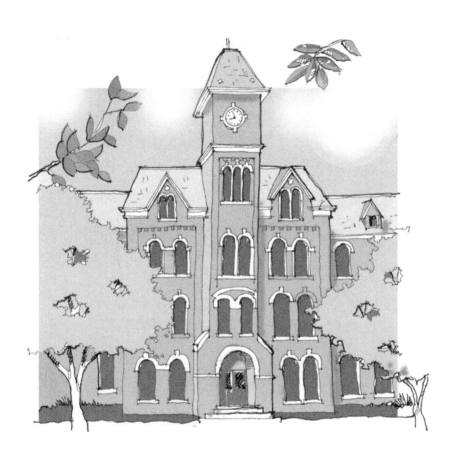

The Summer Session is IN

My husband went to OSU (*The* Ohio State University). I go to OHC. While there are no frat parties at Oncology Hematology Care, the chemo sessions can be a lot of fun. I meet people. I learn things. One visit costs about as much as a semester of college. The really good news is I won't be saddled with $90K in student loans when I "graduate." It's all covered by insurance!

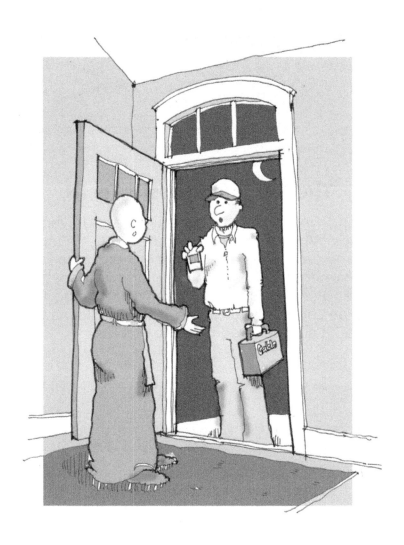

The Cable Repair Window is All Day

Since I was home on Short Term Disability, I finally decided it was time to bundle my cable and internet to save a few bucks. The customer service representative was thrilled to learn my "window" was between 12:01 a.m. and midnight. I think he gave me an extra $1.43 off my monthly bill just for being flexible.

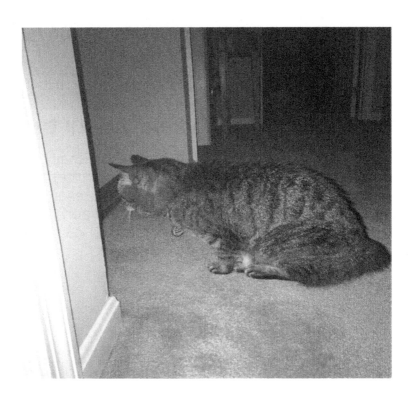

Someone to Watch Over Me

Friends, family and felines are very protective when you have a serious illness. If it were up to Steve, I'd be placed in a bubble to avoid germs and ward off infection. That's another reason I don't sleep. I'm afraid I'll wake up inside an oversized Ziploc bag.

Even the cat is doing her part to protect me. I've been bunking in the upstairs guest bedroom so I don't bother Steve when I get up to use the restroom multiple times a night or to write these perks at 3:45 a.m. Maddy has planted herself outside the bedroom door at the top of the stairs. She won't come into the room. She simply stands like a sentry at Buckingham Palace and I'm Princess Diana (which I am, of course). Who needs the Queen's Guard when you have this little ball of fur?

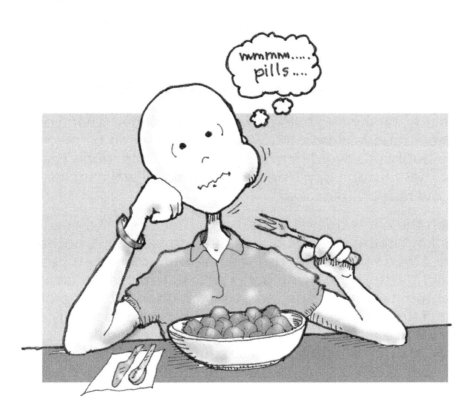

Everything Tastes the Same

This can be a sad side effect from chemo. Pills taste like pills. Honey Nut Cheerios taste like pills. The cardboard box from the Honey Nut Cheerios tastes like pills. Nothing tastes good... just the same.

On the other hand, this can be a real plus if you have a family member with cancer who happens to be a picky eater. You can feed them anything—even Brussel sprouts. Which by the way, I've always believed got a bad rap. They are delicious. Even as very large, green pills.

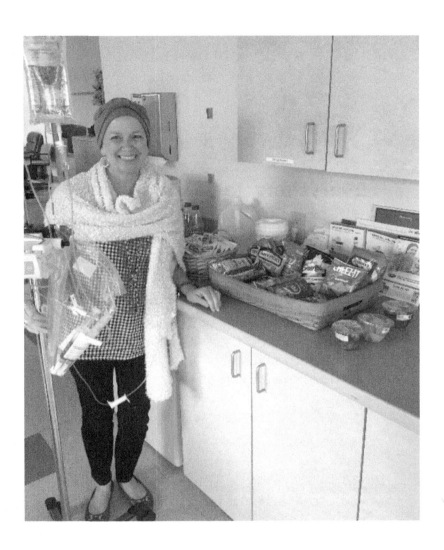

Offsetting Your Co-Pay

Since Steve's heart issue last fall and my diagnosis this spring, we've been fortunate to discover that once you get past the $4,500 per person deductible, we have some fairly decent health insurance. I am just slightly disappointed that my timing was off. Had we coordinated our illnesses, we wouldn't have had to meet the deductible twice in seven months and I'd already have the money to pay for my celebratory post-treatment, cancer-free Viking River Cruise.

The good news is I've figured out a way to outsmart the system. We have a $100 co-pay for my office visits, but free drinks and snacks are available during the chemo treatments. Since Steve goes with me, we can easily each consume $50 worth of bottled water, soft drinks, Cheez-Its, granola bars, nuts and Smart Pop in less than six hours. Boom!

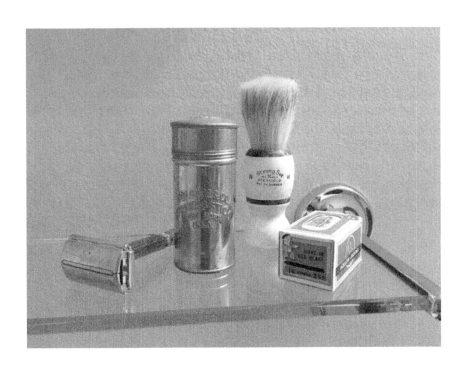

No More Razors

I'm obsessive-compulsive and have shaved my legs every single day since I was 14 years old. *Even in the winter.* That said, a month into treatment I decided to do an experiment and not shave. While I lost the hair on my head, I still have my eyelashes and eyebrows. I was curious as to what was happening with my underarms and shins. I'm on day three of no shaving and everything is still as smooth as a baby's bottom. I spoke to a cancer survivor last week and she said her underarm hair never grew back. Life is good!

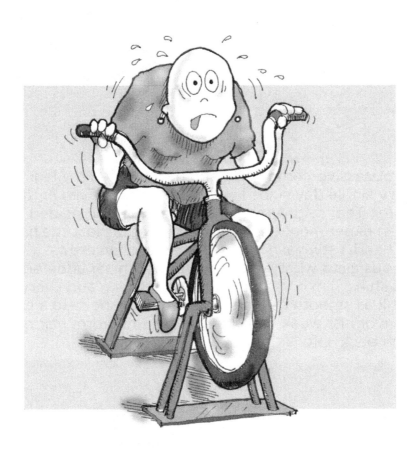

Free Cancer Wellness Program

I joined a fitness class designed specifically for cancer patients to help with muscular strength, endurance and flexibility. Between the cancer, the chemo and the trainer, I'm now thoroughly convinced someone is trying to kill me.

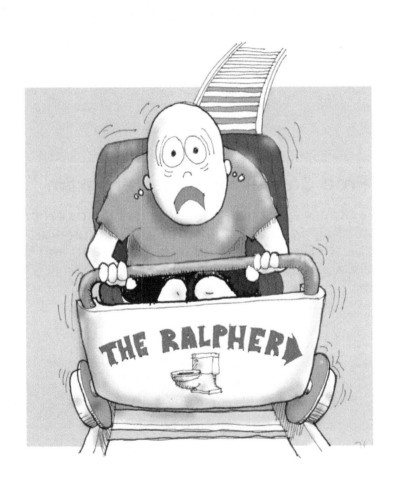

Wild Rides

If you enjoy roller coasters, you'll love cancer. Thrills! Chills! Twists! Turns! Screaming! Puking! Yep, cancer can be all of that and more! Fortunately, I have a cast-iron stomach and have avoided the puking part, but I've had my fair share of ups and downs. For example:

UP

Dr. Chua (smiling and waving two pieces of paper): "Did you see the PET scan results? No cancer! Just like I said it would happen. The remaining treatments will shrink the lymph nodes."

Me (patting my mid-section): "So, does that mean I'll have a flat tummy when this is all said and done?"

DOWN

Dr. Chua: "No, that's just fat."

Me: *"Dang."*

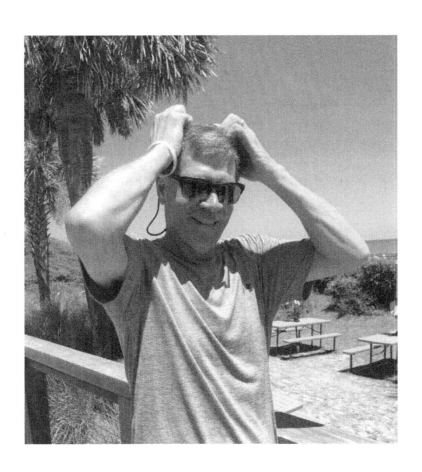

No No-See-Ums!

Summer vacations in the South are a lot of fun despite the blistering sun, alligators, jellyfish, copperheads and palmetto bugs large enough to saddle up and ride. I was feeling good after my third treatment, so Steve and I decided to drive to Hilton Head for some R&R (like I wasn't getting enough of THAT). While enjoying a frozen virgin piña colada at the beach bar, I looked over to see Steve doing some crazy dance and scratching like a hound. Ah... the dreaded No-See-Um—a ferocious, minuscule biting fly that likes to get in your hair and attack your scalp. Thanks to my lack o' hair and bullet-proof chemo beanie, I wasn't getting bit at all. Another perk, indeed!

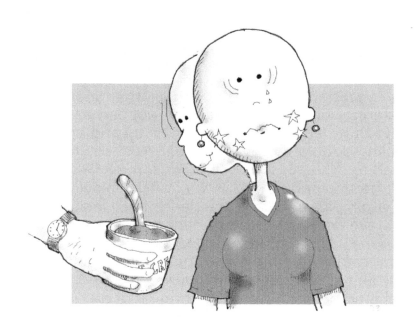

Mucositis

My oncologist mentioned that chemo can cause painful ulcers in the mouth known as oral mucositis. I became lax in my baking soda/salt-water rinse routine and consequently developed sores inside my cheek and under my tongue. Dr. Chua was right—they are painful. If you do not have initials behind your name like M.D., PhD or D.O., you really should heed the advice of someone who does.

Because I'm an idiot, it now smarts to talk. That's where the perk for your spouse or significant other comes in. I went three whole hours without complaining, nagging or saying a word. Steve said it gave new meaning to "peaceful vacation."

It also hurts to eat. The good news is that just before this all went down, I discovered chocolate toasted coconut ice cream. Ice cream eases the pain for breakfast, lunch and dinner, so I guess you could say the inflammation is somewhat of a perk for me, too.

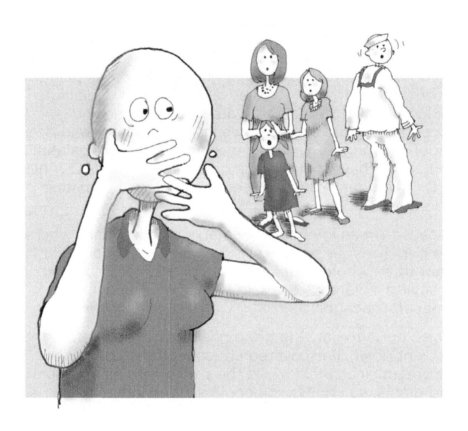

Four Letter Words

S#%t. D@!!!n. Even the occasional F-bomb. When someone has cancer, even the most refined lady or polished gentleman may find cuss words flowing easily out of their potty mouths, especially after discovering sores in said potty mouth, or on the fourth day of actually not s#%ting. The good news is that even the most proper person will simply look at you and nod in agreement. After all, you have "The Big C." Just don't make a habit of it unless you are a sailor.

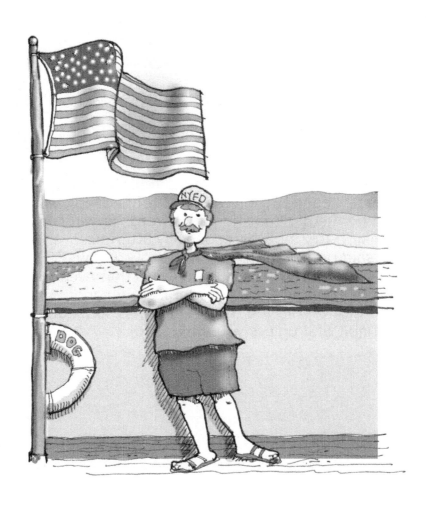

Real Superheroes

Having no hair as a woman is typically a giveaway that you have cancer. It can also be a terrific conversation starter. While in Hilton Head, I was on the Salty Dog Happy Hour Cruise (not *my* boat, but at least a boat) where Bill, a kind man from New York City, was enjoying some special time with his family. His stepdaughter had just gotten engaged and everyone was in great spirits. Bill came to the rail and we struck up a conversation. He asked me about my cancer and shared that he had been a firefighter at Ground Zero during 9/11. As a result of his rescue efforts during that time, he had been battling multiple myeloma the last four years. He had the most amazing attitude, and although he would never be cured, he was making the most out of every day. I was in awe of his positivity and humble demeanor.

Bill did not play professional sports. We've not seen him on the big screen. He doesn't wear a cape (at least he didn't that evening). But Bill is a REAL superhero and one of the most inspiring people I'll ever meet. God bless America and God bless Bill!

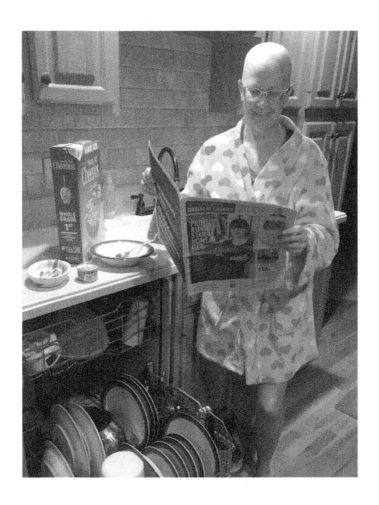

Multi-Tasking

I've found myself slowing down a bit. I've also found myself with more free time than ever before. I realized at breakfast this morning that I could actually sit down at the countertop island and enjoy my cereal and MiraLAX-infused orange juice without having to simultaneously unload the dishwasher, feed the cat and read the newspaper. What was formerly one task has now become four separate events. Who knew?

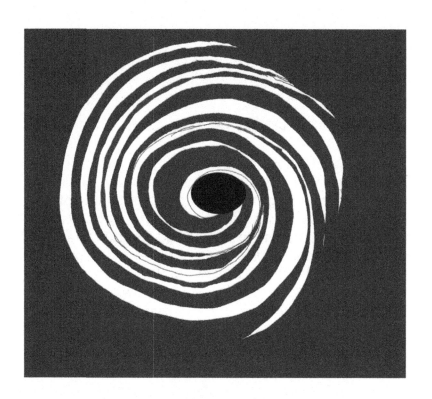

Bad Days

There will be bad days. Or bad nights. Or both. It's okay to wallow in the black hole for a brief moment. But only for a moment. Please try to find something good about each day even if you can only say, "Well, at least no fingers or toes fell off while I was sleeping."

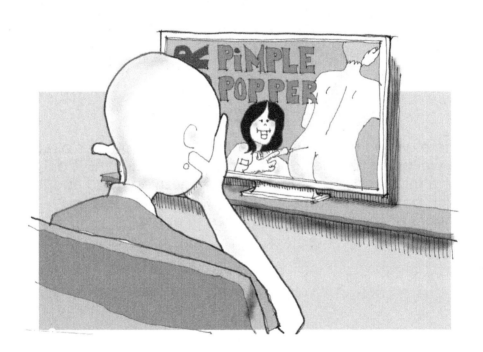

Reality TV

At some point you will find yourself engrossed—emphasis on *gross*—in an episode of *Dr. Pimple Popper*. Watch it. It will make you feel better about all of the poking and prodding that is happening to your own body. Hopefully, your doctor will not be removing something from your backside that looks like it came from the science fiction movie *The Blob*.

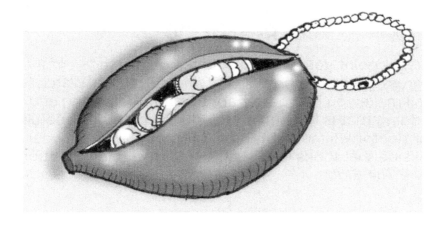

You Won't Need a Chiropractor

You've heard horror stories about people who have been so far out of alignment they needed surgery from years of carrying purses, backpacks or briefcases that were far too heavy. I have good news! As you become weaker, your wallet becomes lighter. Watch the medical bills pour in and by the end of your treatment, you won't even need a wallet. A simple coin purse like the one you carried in grade school will sufficiently hold all of your net worth.

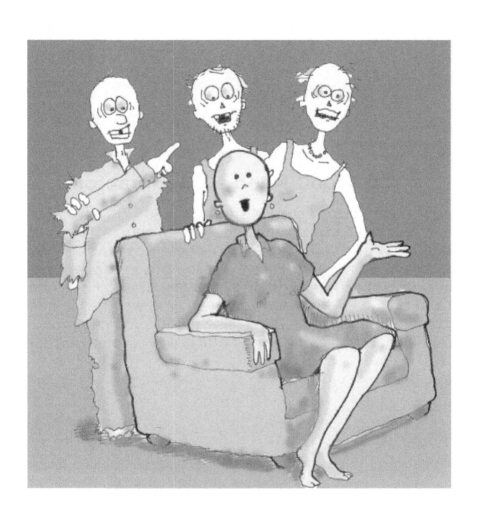

I See Dead People

Well, I don't really *see* dead people. I do *talk* to them, though. You may also find yourself having full conversations with your deceased parents, grandparents, in-laws, friends and other relatives, asking them to pull a few strings "up there." Trust me, it *will* happen at least once.

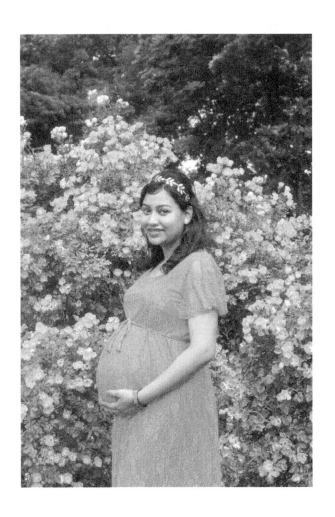

Eat Whatever You Want

It's important to keep up your strength and maintain your weight when going through treatment. A good way to do this is live by the policy, "If it smells good, eat it." And remember, pasta salad, a pickle and an ice cream cone can be the new Breakfast of Champions!

All the rules that apply to your pregnant friends now apply to you.

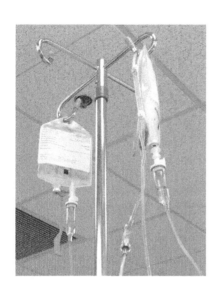
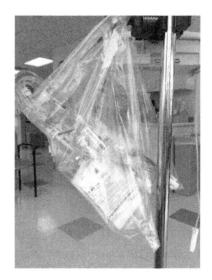

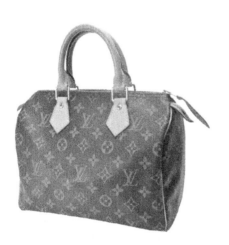
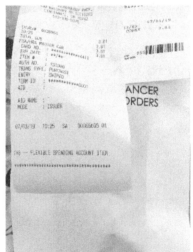

Games to Pass the Time

This one is called "Which Bag is the Most Expensive?"

Hint: It's not the Louis Vuitton!

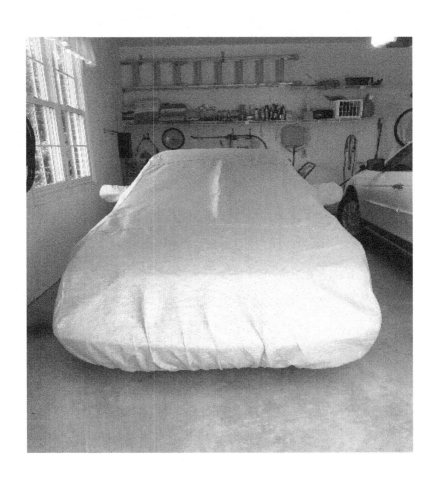

Drive the Convertible

When we moved Mom into a nursing home in the mid-1990s, we began to go through her things. Nothing saddened me more than the gift box on the top shelf of her closet that contained hand-embroidered pillowcases with a wedding card dated June 7, 1959 tucked inside. She had been saving them for a special occasion.

Isn't every day special?

Uncover the convertible and drive it.

Serve Hamburger Helper on your fine china.

Light the candles.

Use the embroidered pillowcases, for goodness sake!

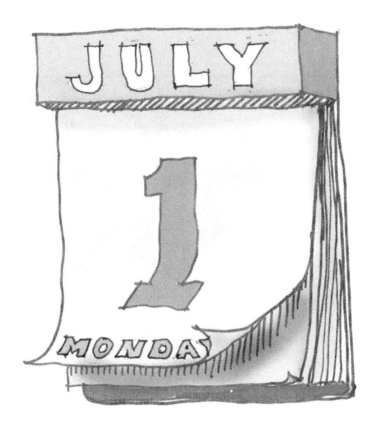

*"Whether you think you can,
or you think you can't, you're right."*

—Henry Ford

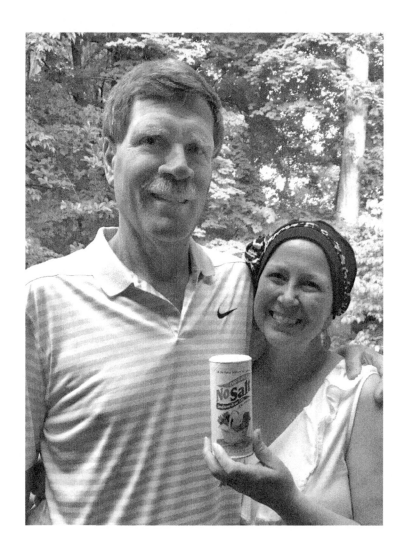

Becoming Closer to Your Significant Other

After more than three decades of marriage, I didn't think I could love my husband more, but I do. Both of our health issues this past year have brought us closer to the realization that someday, one of us will be living without the other. Neither wants that to happen anytime soon.

When Steve had his heart trouble, my form of love came via way of "The Salt Nazi." I gave away anything with more than 400 mg of sodium and immediately tore out every casserole recipe from my cookbooks that included a can of soup. I've watched his sodium intake like a hawk. I added an addendum to our wedding vows: "I promise to prepare and feed you only heart-healthy foods, from this day forward, as long as we both shall live."

When I got sick, Steve became more protective, more emotional, more romantic and more affectionate. I often find a card on the nightstand when I awake in the morning, or he hands it to me personally with a tear in his eye. He makes sure no one enters the house without removing their shoes and using the jumbo bottle of hand sanitizer. He tucks me into bed each night and snuggles with me for a full fifteen minutes without me having to beg. He tells me that being bald doesn't matter and that he loves me. And I believe him.

Being married to my best friend has been the biggest perk of all. I'm one of the lucky ones. I didn't need to get cancer to know this. I knew it all along, it's just a bit more real now.

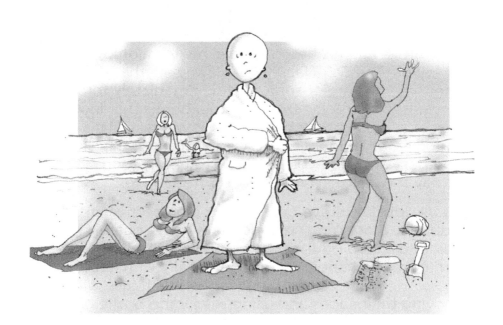

Morbid Thoughts

Holidays might have you thinking things like, "What if this were my last Fourth of July?" I'd want to go out with a BIG BANG of course! You don't need cancer to have these thoughts. You never know when your number is up. I don't want my last day to be anytime soon, so I'm following doctor's orders as well as making a point to make every day count and every day last (again prednisone helps here, because you can maximize your days by staying awake for 72 straight hours).

July fifth happens to be National Bikini Day. Sadly, for me that ship sailed years ago. I'll celebrate the day in my full-coverage tankini. I don't want some old geezer at the pool seeing me in a thong and having a heart attack. I'd hate to be responsible for someone else's last day.

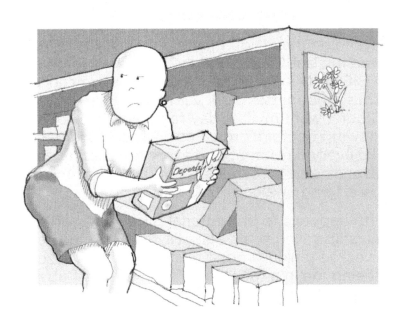

Consider Wetting the Bed

I know this is not a perk, but my thoughts were so ridiculous I had to write them down. Sometime after your fourth round of chemo, drinking more than thirty gallons of water a day, when you have to pee for the fourth time at 3:34 a.m., you will seriously consider wetting the bed, *on purpose*. You are sleeping in the upstairs guest room so as not to disturb your spouse. The mattress was purchased three decades ago anyway. Besides, you can always wash the sheets and your pajama bottoms, right? So why not let loose? Of course, you don't. You make that thirty-four-step trek to the bathroom and pee for what seems like thirty-four minutes. You flush the toilet not twice, but three times for good measure, then head back to bed and seriously consider purchasing Depends tomorrow.

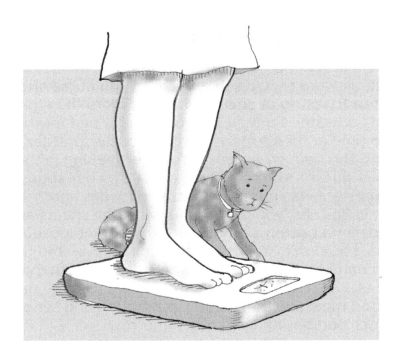

Weight Loss

Unfortunately, my timing was a bit off on this too, as cancer can be an easy-to-follow weight loss program. A year earlier I stepped on the scale and realized I had gained a bit of weight since I got married. I recalled something my former boss had said to me back in 1987—a woman gains a pound a year for every year she is married. My scale clearly indicated I was married for thirty-six years, but it had only been thirty-one. Time to go on a diet! I selected WW (formerly known as Weight Watchers) and it was a fantastic program. I lost twenty pounds within six months and kept it off. I felt great! That is, until I got cancer and started losing more weight. Had I only waited fourteen more months, I could have skipped the meetings, counting points and downloading the app. Figures!

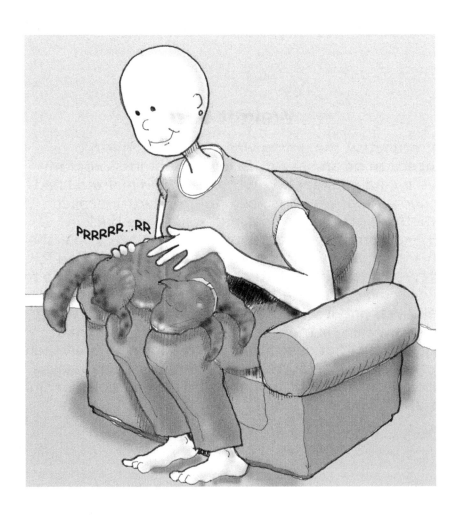

Pets

Animals seem to know when something is wrong. Our cat, Maddy, is no exception. For nine years, Maddy has been "Daddy's Girl", but not anymore! Of late, it's my lap she prefers. I'm now the recipient of the majority of special head butts and massages. She's another reason I'm not getting anything accomplished and I'm loving every minute of it.

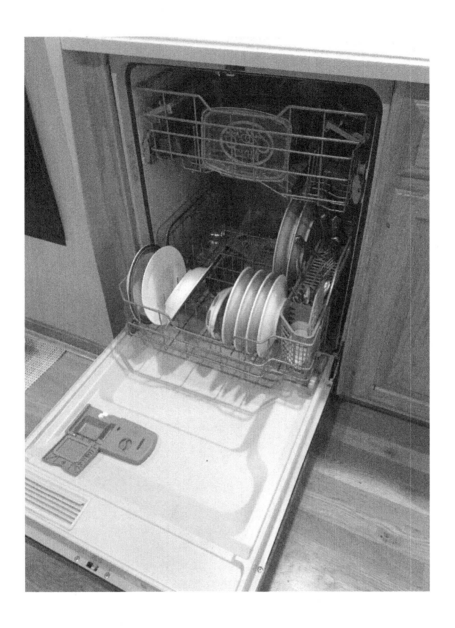

Prioritizing Time

Small projects can become big deals. Tackle them accordingly. As your energy is depleted and the only project you are up for is unloading the lower rack of the dishwasher, do it and be proud of your accomplishments!

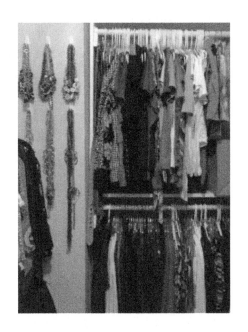

Before cancer

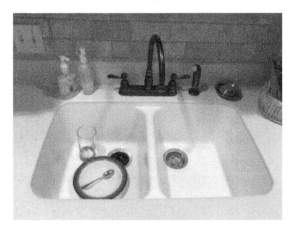

After cancer

Becoming Less Obsessive-Compulsive

It's no secret, I have OCD. My husband is even worse. He's exactly what my mother wished on me. Before cancer, I could not leave for work until the house was in complete order, including everything in my closet organized by color. After cancer, I actually started leaving my breakfast dishes in the sink and was shocked to learn that when I came back from my morning walk, the world had not ended, the house had not crumbled and the dishes were still there.

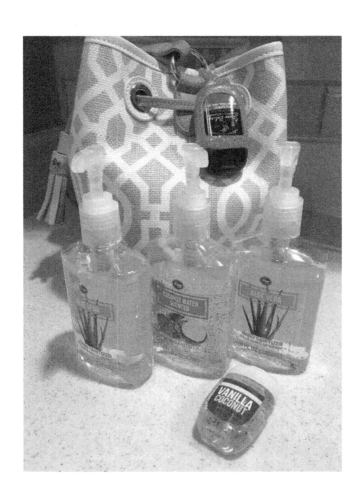

Stock Options

It's possible to bulk up your portfolio again by purchasing stock in companies that produce hand-sanitizer. No further explanation needed.

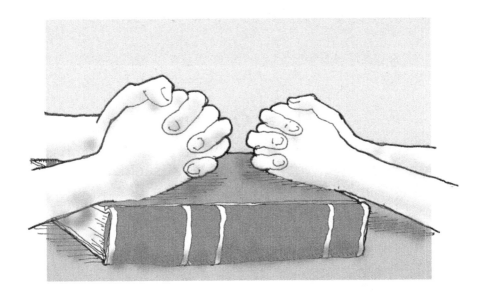

Resilience

On days when a train seems to have run you over, don't quit. There are too many people from the prayer chain counting on you to show the world the power of prayer can overcome anything. PROVE. THEM. RIGHT!

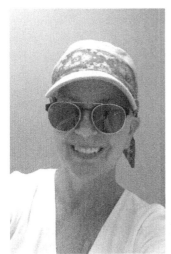
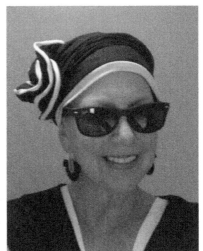
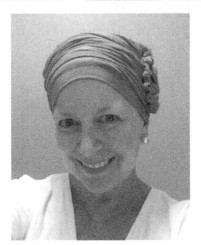

Hats

I love hats. Going to the Kentucky Derby and wearing one as large as a patio umbrella has always been on my bucket list. Since I used to wear my hair short, I never felt comfortable in a hat because I thought it made me look bald. Now that my head is as smooth as a cue ball, I'm not comfortable without one!

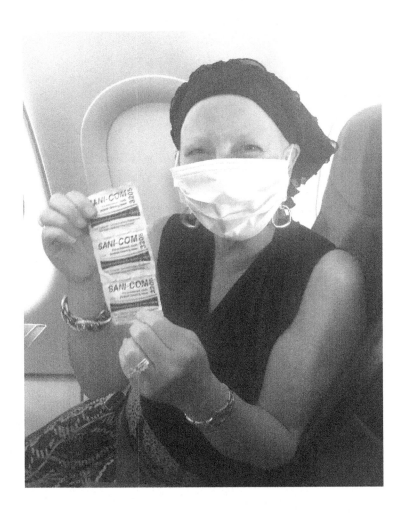

In-Flight Service

While you have to pay for drinks, peanuts and carry-on bags in addition to a seat on low-cost carriers, I discovered that if you wear a hospital mask on the plane, flight attendants are very attentive. Five packets of sanitary wipes plus a complimentary barf bag in case chemo makes you nauseated add up to some great freebie perks!

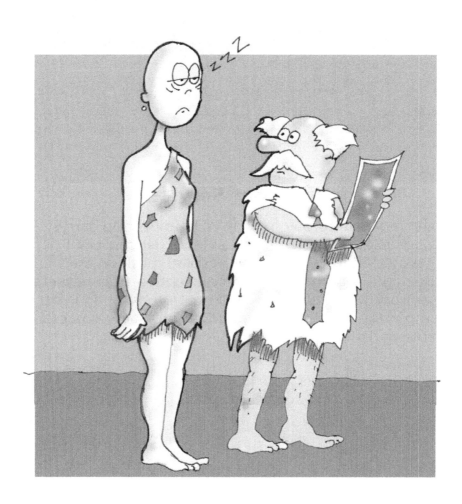

Prednisone Again

I'm back on the five pills for five days regimen. Does anyone recall the *Flintstones* episode where Wilma, Betty and Barney thought they had to keep Fred awake for 72 hours or he would die? I'm Fred! I'll have my *Perks of Having Cancer* book completed by my next treatment—two rounds ahead of schedule and I'll be starting on the sequel: *The Perils of Prednisone!*

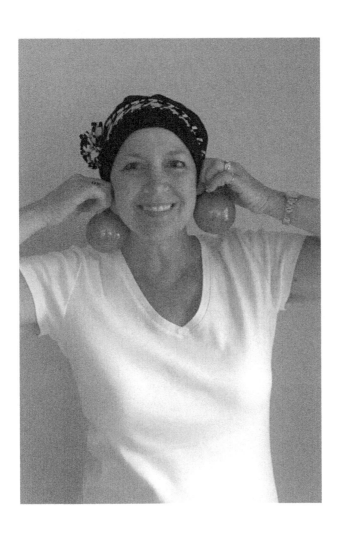

Earrings

You will become convinced that the bigger the earrings, the less likely folks will notice you are wearing a chemo beanie because you are bald. I actually considered wearing Christmas ornaments to a recent family picnic. Fortunately, Steve nixed the idea before I made a complete fool of myself.

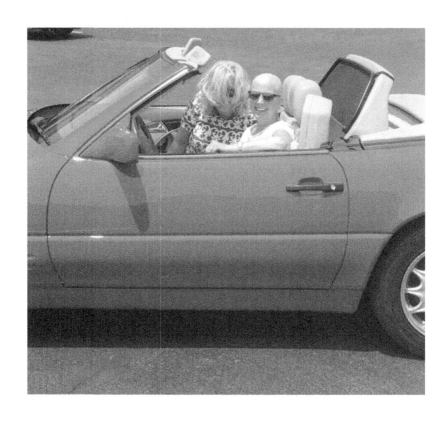

Hassle Free Convertible Rides

Lack of hair in a ragtop equates to a safer, more comfortable ride. No chance of eating your own locks, getting strands in your eyes or stuck in your lip gloss. Additionally, the aerodynamics from your slick, bald noggin may allow for improved gas mileage.

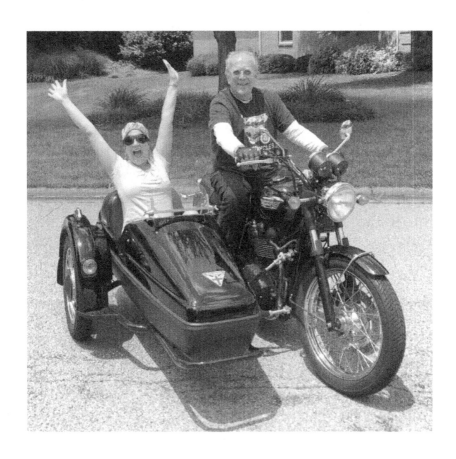

Be Adventurous

Decades ago, I went to see a fortune teller. She told me that I would live a very long life. I took that to heart and over the years took risks I probably shouldn't have, believing I was somewhat invincible. Cancer proved that I'm not. But cancer is NOT going to beat me. I want to leave this world doing something I love; therefore, I'll continue to take risks. Tim McGraw was right—you should live like you are dying. Life is much more fun that way.

If you can still hear your fears, shift the gears!

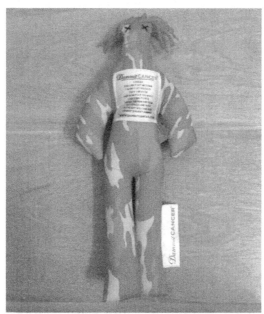

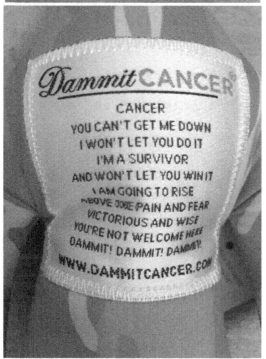

Dolls

You are never too old to play with dolls.

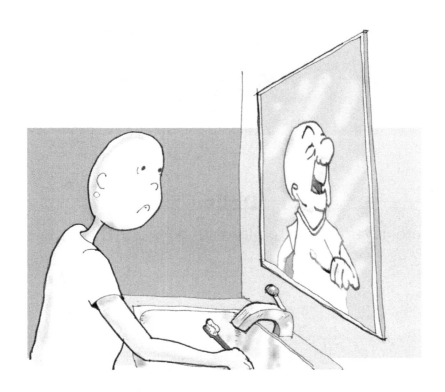

On Being Bald

As you pass a mirror, the shock of seeing Mr. Magoo staring back at you starts to get easier as time goes on.

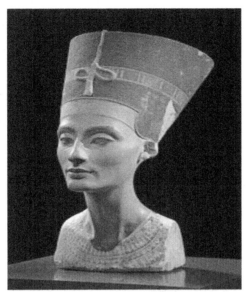

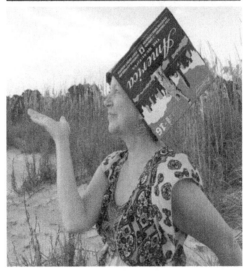

Creative Head Coverings

After wearing the same six chemo beanies every day for six weeks, a recent exhibit at the Cincinnati Museum Center featuring "Egypt: The Time of The Pharaohs," had me yearning for something a bit different. I tried to recreate Queen Nefertiti's headdress out of a Budweiser carton, but it didn't come off the way I had hoped. I guess I'm not cut out to be a queen. I'll settle for Princess Diana.

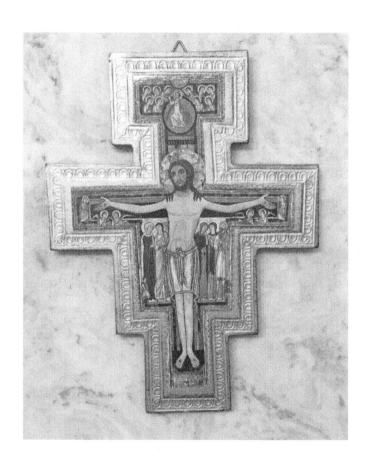

More God Winks

The daily Mass I attend is held in the small Day Chapel at St. Columban. I had rarely been inside the chapel prior to my illness and was immediately drawn to this cross. It's so vibrant and colorful, with incredible detail. I knew nothing about it—it was just something I found to be beautiful.

When my sister-in-law returned from Rome, I learned she had brought us a cross to hang in our home—the San Damiano Cross—which is *the same cross I've been admiring the last few months at my church!* The cross is named for one of the patron saints of healing—St. Damian. Pam selected it because Jesus was looking up and hopeful, versus most crosses that show Him with His head hanging down. Pam also brought me a two-page sheet of explanations—the shape (the key to heaven), the colors (red, the color of blood and life; black, the color of death; gold for the regal Holy Trinity), the hand of God (so we feel blessed as we pray), the eyes of Jesus (following us with the look of love), shells (symbols of the beach and eternity) plus a clarification of the various figures depicted.

It's no coincidence that Pam selected this piece to bring me peace.

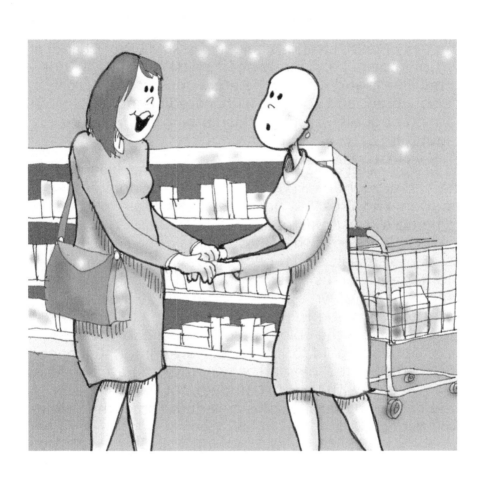

Humble and Kind

For the third time in as many months, a complete stranger made my day. The stories are all similar: a cancer survivor reaching out to a stranger who obviously has cancer.

Last evening, as I turned the corner in search of low sodium salad dressing, a woman stopped in front of my grocery cart, looked me in the eye, smiled, and said quite loudly, "You can do it!" She didn't look familiar, but I was unsure if my chemo brain was just failing to recall her name or if she truly was a stranger. She then stepped around my cart and before I could stop her, she wrapped her arms around me and said again, "You can do it!" She explained that she was a breast cancer survivor and wished me well. I shared with her that my last treatment was coming up soon and yes, I knew I could do it, but I so appreciated her reaching out. I really did.

I honestly wish there were more people like her in this world—strangers willing to share the love instead of hate. I don't know if this woman was Democrat or Republican, if she supported gun control or had an NRA sticker on her car, if she wanted to build a wall or was harboring an illegal immigrant in her basement, was atheist or Christian, gay or straight. What I do know is that she was kind. And that humbled me.

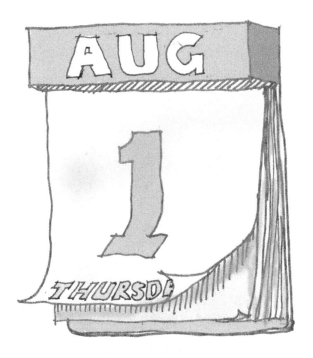

"You gain strength, courage and confidence by every experience in which you really stop to look fear in the face. You are able to say to yourself, 'I lived through this horror. I can take the next thing that comes along...'

"We must do the things we think we cannot."

—Eleanor Roosevelt

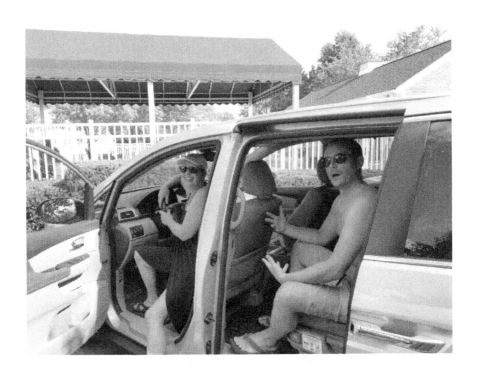

Grand Theft Auto

It may have been the chemo brain.

It may have been the hot sun.

It may have been a flashback to the Savannah/Hilton Head International Airport where I have rented many an automobile from National Car Rental's Emerald Aisle, where you select any car from under the green awning.

Regardless, I stole a vehicle.

Tammy had driven her silver Toyota Rav4 with the nice wheels to the community pool. When we ran low on drinks, I offered to run home to refill the cooler. There were three silver SUV's with nice rims in the lot. I took the middle one. I didn't notice it was a Honda Odyssey with three rows and a car seat in the back. I got in, pushed the starter button and drove home.

I had never met my neighbor Nelson before. I now know him well after stealing his car to replenish my friend's alcohol stash. Fortunately, he's a kind young man who decided not to press charges. He asked if I was drunk. I only wish I had been.

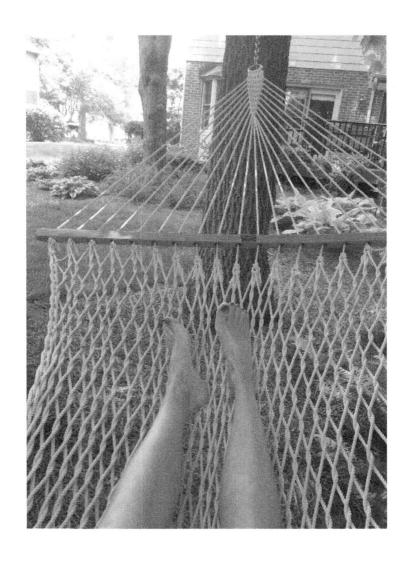

Rediscovering the Hammock

We've had a hammock in our backyard for nearly thirty years. I can count on one hand how many times I've been in the "Nappy Thing," as my niece used to call it (i.e. thing to take a nap in). Until recently. Now, weather permitting, it's become part of my daily routine and an extension of my backside. I can spend hours in the thing. Of course, the main reason is that it's actually easier to get *into* the Nappy Thing than it is to get *out of* the Nappy Thing. I feel like a big ole' crab caught in a net.

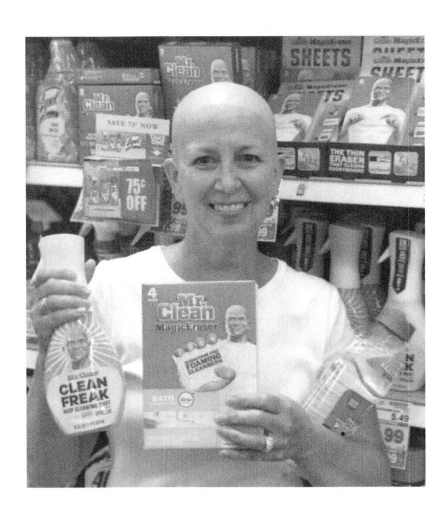

Extra Income

Proctor & Gamble held tryouts for "Mr. Clean" a couple of years ago and I hear the gig paid $20,000. I think it's time for "*Mrs.* Clean" to plug the Magic Eraser, don't you?

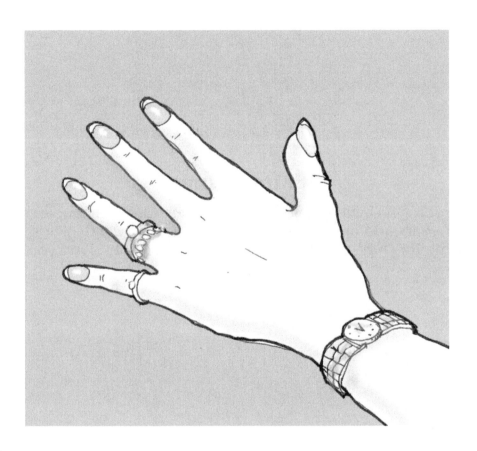

Long Nails

For the first time in my life, I have pretty fingernails without the help of acrylic or gel. All I had to do to get them was *absolutely nothing*. Seriously, if you do *absolutely nothing* but lay in the hammock and watch your nails grow... your nails will grow. I'm not working; therefore, I'm not loading and unloading trucks for events. With the meal train, I'm not cooking. Someone else cleans my toilets, shower, and the litterbox. I'm considering hiring a lady's maid like Anna Bates from *Downton Abbey*. I certainly don't want to risk chipping my polish by dressing myself!

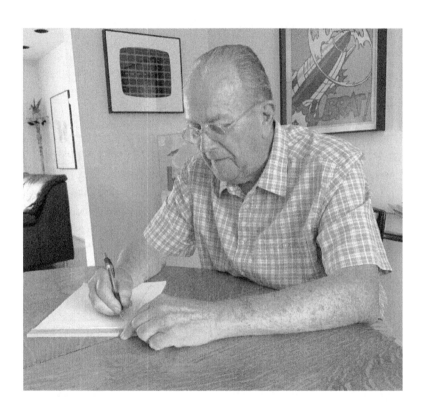

Loved Ones Love to Help Out

They may even write a perk for you when you find your tears are flowing more freely than your creative juices. I received the following text from my birth father. It also explains where I get my sense of humor:

I thought of a perk you can look forward to.

When I call any medical provider to make an appointment, they naturally ask my date of birth. When they hear my birth year is 1943, they ask me:

"Can you stand?"

"Do you need a wheelchair?"

"Do you have a pacemaker?"

"How about visual impairments?"

After I answer "No" to all their questions, I feel so good I consider canceling the appointment. I've started calling occasionally for no reason, just to make myself feel better.

Love, Big Poppa

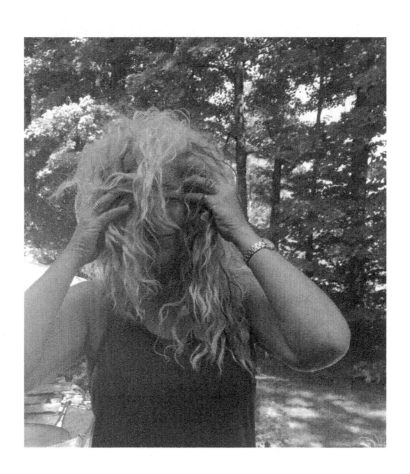

Free Wigs

The problem with free wigs is they might not look anything like your hair prior to cancer in color, texture, style or length. Therefore, you get what you pay for. But if you are over 55 years of age (which I am), you'll take anything for free. All senior citizens take free stuff—*even if they don't want it or need it*. I believe it's a law in 37 states and the District of Columbia.

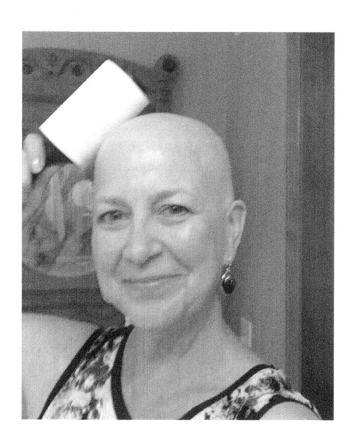

New Uses for Everyday Objects

Despite having my head shaved, there are still some patches of bristle atop the noodle. Just because the hair is short doesn't mean it's stopped falling out. Plus, it itches like crazy. When I scratched my head over the bathroom sink, it looked like Steve had just cleaned out his electric razor. I had the lint roller on the counter to remove some cat hair from my black leggings and thought, "Why not?" I rolled the thing across my head a few times, collected several hundred pieces of stubble—and my sink remained sparkling clean. Who knew?!?! 3M will thank me after my book is published as I'm sure this technique will result in dramatically increased sales of Scotch Brite rollers.

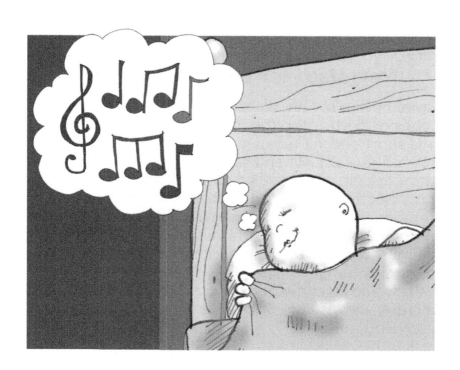

Untapped Potential

One sleepless night you may discover long hidden talents deep within your core. I'm now a songwriter. I call this little ditty, *Zoning Out on Prednisone.* If you've ever been prescribed prednisone, feel free to sing along!

Poppin' orange chalky pills,

To cure all my cancer ills,

I'm zoning out on prednisone!

I'm no longer lazy,

But they makin' me crazy,

I'm zoning out on prednisone!

Sweatin' like a stuck hog,

Meaner than a junkyard dog,

I'm zoning out on prednisone!

Staying up all night,

Eating every single bite,

I'm zoning out on prednisone!

Happy I'm not gaining weight,

I'd give anything to sleep in late,

I'm zoning out on prednisone!

My skin is peeling off my head,

It's better off than bein' dead,

I'm zoning out on prednisone!

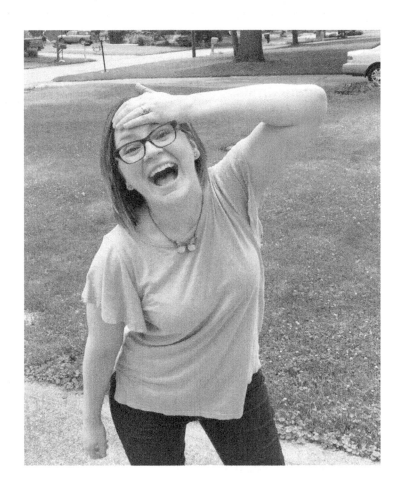

People Say The Darndest Things

At the end of a recent visit from my sweet co-worker Kristin, she said, "Well, it's getting late, I'd better get out of your hair." I immediately started cracking up. She looked at me in my chemo beanie, realized what she had said, and was appalled. I don't know what was more hilarious... the comment or the look on her face. Poor thing!

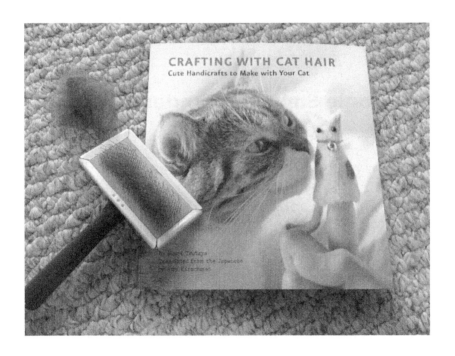

Bizarre Gifts

You may find yourself the recipient of some strange presents. Toward the end of your medical leave, you may actually consider using them because you are JUST. THAT. BORED.

If someone actually was able to print and sell a book about craft projects from cat hair, I am pretty sure I can compile these crazy perks into a book and sell a few copies.

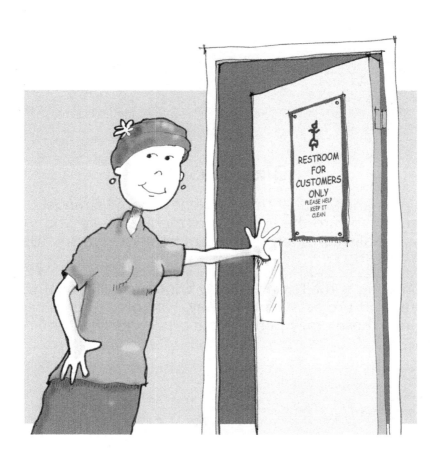

Pulling the Cancer Card

The "cancer card" is great to redeem for back rubs, excusing yourself from housework, oversleeping, getting into any bathroom even if you are not a patron—the possibilities are endless. I recommend, however, dealing out the card sparingly as I've discovered it tends to wear thin with overuse.

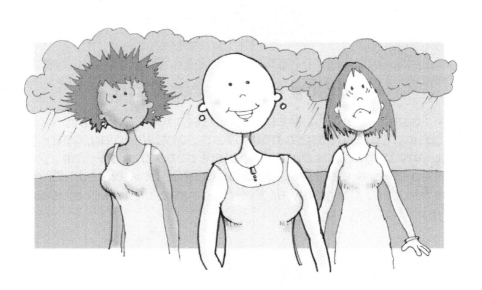

Humidity

When the forecast calls for 100 percent humidity, you no longer have to worry about flat hair (for those of us who used to have fine hair) or frizz (for those of you who used to have thick locks).

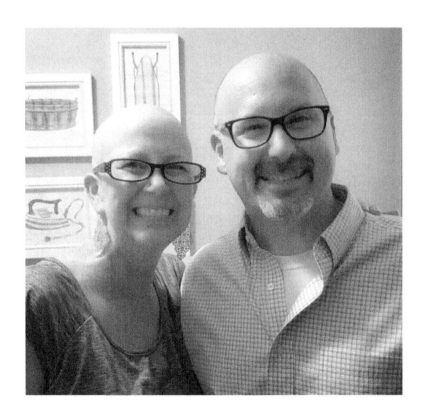

Twins

I've heard some people look like their pets. Others look like their spouses. I now happen to look like my friend, Jeff. If he had earrings and I had a goatee, you wouldn't be able to tell us apart. Oh, brother!

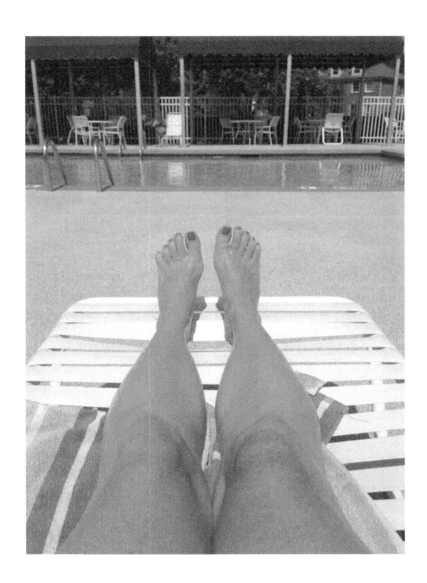

Solitude

If your chemo treatments coincide with summer, by mid-August you will find yourself to be the only person poolside at 11 a.m. on a Thursday. Don't forget to take your sunscreen because no one will be there for you to ask to borrow some. Heaven on earth!

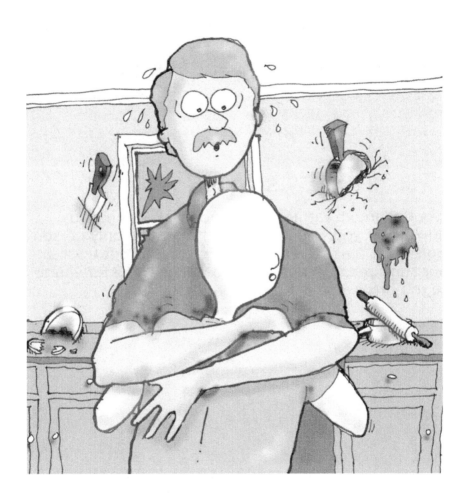

Forgiveness

Even the kindest person will have a rough day and snap at their husband or, worse yet, throw a skillet across the kitchen at his head. As long as you miss, he will just hug you and say, "Honey, I understand. I can't imagine how hard this is for you."

God bless him.

I love him so much.

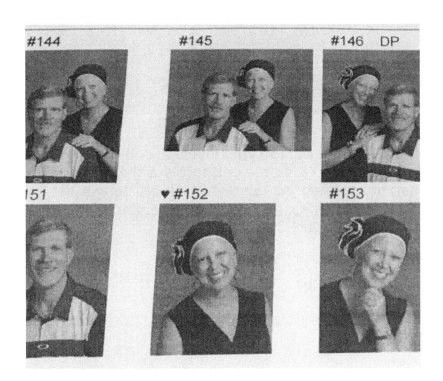

Unique Family Photos

I'm fairly certain I'm the only woman who is a.) wearing a hat and b.) bald as an eagle sitting for the 160-year anniversary edition of our church directory. Oh well, I should have locks again by the 165th.

Note: The photographer insisted on the Glamour Shot/ Chin Grab pose. Those are so cheesy! He convinced me to do it only after he said it would hide two of my three chins.

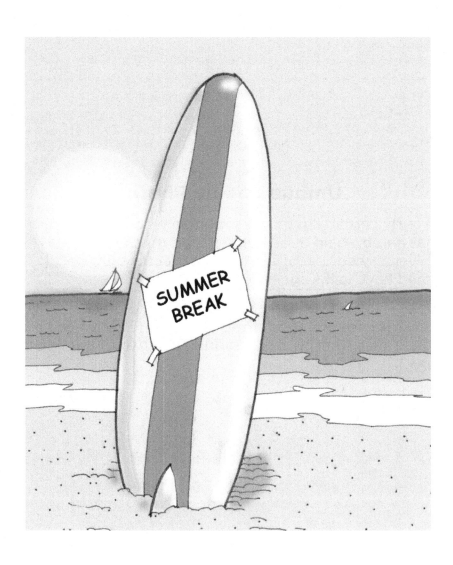

Summer Break

I may not have been as positive and upbeat about my situation had my diagnosis occurred during the gray gloom of a Cincinnati winter. Sunshine and warmth fuel my soul; therefore, I *love* summer! And I've not had the entire season off school or work since I was 15 years old. I realize I've enjoyed the exact same activities I did more than forty years ago:

- Staying in bed until 10 a.m.

- Laying around on the couch for hours

- Eating whatever I want, whenever I want, and not gaining weight

- Enjoying time in my backyard reading

- Searching for four-leaf clovers

- Receiving a small allowance

- Letting others drive me around town

- Spending time with friends (or *not* on the days I was "grounded" inside the house, LOL!)

- Lounging by the pool

- Listening to cicadas during the day

- Watching lightning bugs in the evening

- Staying up late to watch TV (back then, I'd watch Johnny Carson followed by an old movie with mom until 3:30 a.m.; now, making it through the 9 p.m. *Antiques Roadshow* on PBS is considered late for me)

Yet like that summer many, many years ago, all good things must come to an end. My "vacation" is officially over the Tuesday after Labor Day when I return to work. Just like the good old days when school didn't start until September.

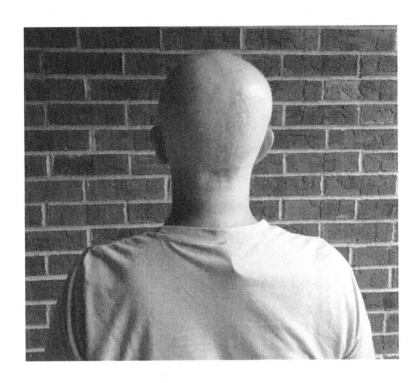

Compliments

An interesting evolution of random, somewhat flattering remarks received throughout my life:

In my late teens: "Nice butt."

In my early twenties: "Nice boobs."

In my mid-thirties: "Nice legs."

In my early forties: "Nice hair."

In my late fifties: "Well, at least you have a nicely shaped head."

My, how times—and body parts—have changed. Sigh.

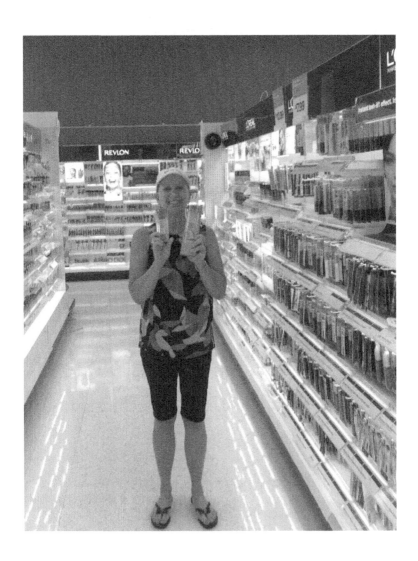

Isle/Aisle of Hope

The ball cap I am wearing is from Isle of Hope, a small island off the Georgia coast near Savannah. Now that I've finished chemo, I sailed into another "Aisle" of Hope at Target, where I purchased eyelash serum and strengthening shampoo. I am looking forward to applying mascara to more than a dozen lashes and combing a full head of hair again soon!

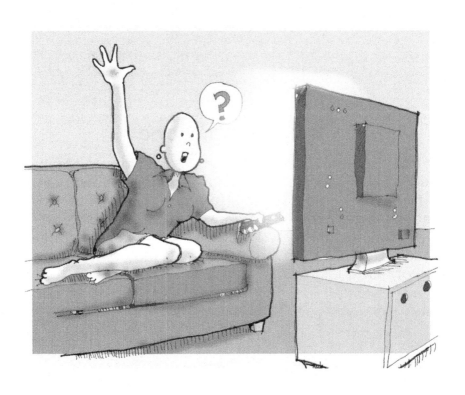

Daytime Television

If you enjoy watching hundreds of commercials for medications that you should "ask your doctor about," or if you've been injured in an accident and are searching for a lawyer, daytime TV is for you. If only I had a dollar for each of these commercials I've watched since last spring, I could pay off the medical bills from doctors of whom I asked too many questions.

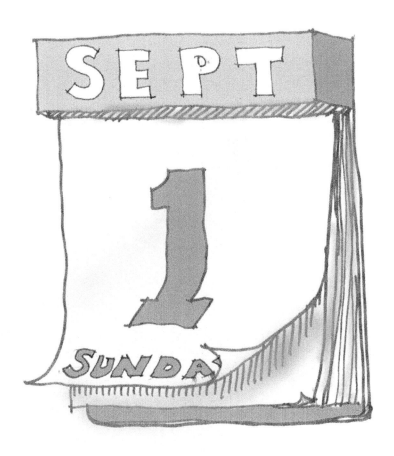

"All our infirmities, whatever they are, are just opportunities for God to display his gracious work in us."

—C. H. Spurgeon

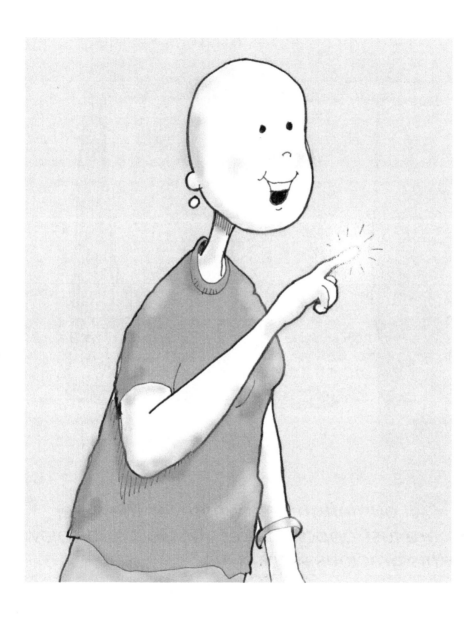

E.T.

Earlier in my journey I bragged about having eyelashes and nice nails. I spoke too soon. The last round of chemo stole my last bit of femininity. My fingernails are now brittle. My bald head is peeling. My eyebrows are thin and I'm down to nine eyelashes. Since May I've gone from looking like Pitbull to looking like an alien. The good news is my treatments are now behind me and I'm hopeful that everything will soon fill in, strengthen up and grow back.

Although he thought it funny at first, Steve is tiring of me running around the house all wrinkly and naked, pointing my index finger and calling out in a wavering voice, "E.T., phone home."

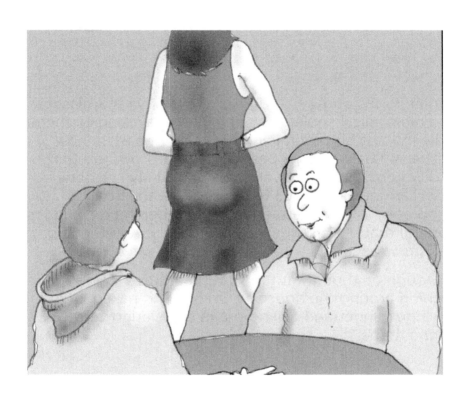

"Can't See the Line, Can You Russ?"

There are so many classic lines by Chevy Chase in *Christmas Vacation.* I love that movie almost as much as I love no lines—no panty lines, yes, but also no lines to wait in. The lack of lines and light traffic will be coming to an end once I return to work. I'm certainly going to miss the ability to grocery shop in the middle of the day in the middle of the week, avoiding the mob of blue personal shopper carts in every aisle. I'll also miss cruising the expressway at times other than rush hour. I'll miss being the only person at the pharmacy drive-thru window. I'll miss the daily half-hour Mass at St. Columban, as now the hour-long Sunday morning Mass seems about a half-hour too long. Most of all, I'll miss Ellen's daily punch lines at 4 p.m. on the couch with the cat on my lap.

Yes, I'll miss a lot of things... but cancer won't be one of them.

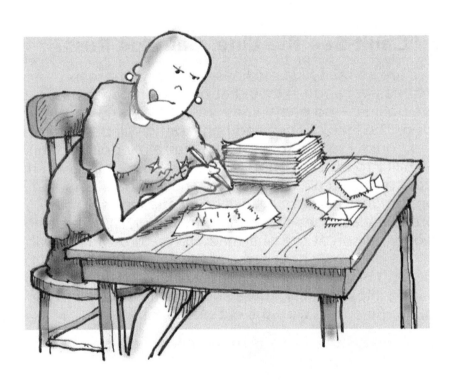

Practicing Penmanship

In the age of computers, penmanship has become a lost art. But with all the insurance paperwork I've completed, as well as thank-you notes written, I've rediscovered handwriting. I've not scribbled out this many A, E, I, O and U's (mostly I.O.U.'s) since second grade. I believe Mrs. Brown would be proud of my work.

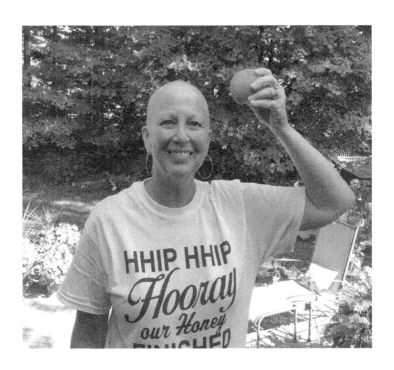

Just Peachy!

I've gone from looking like Pitbull to resembling a fruit with a pit. The peach fuzz indicates my hair is starting to come back.

Now where did I put my comb?

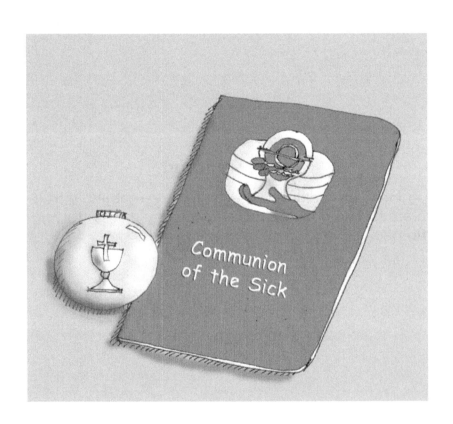

Returns

I returned these items to Father Larry, grateful that I was feeling well enough each week to attend church and that I'm no longer sick and homebound.

Thanks be to God!

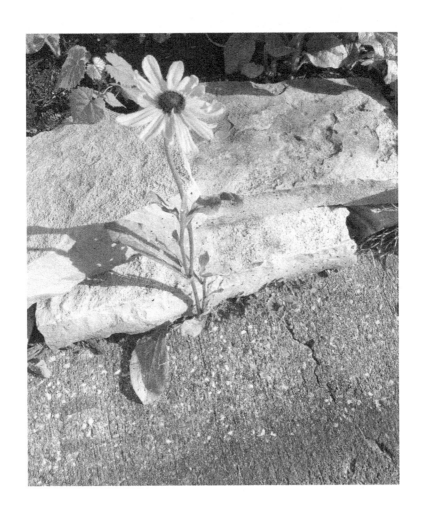

Extraordinary Feats

While awaiting the results of a PET scan, it seems I have the ability to hold my breath for up to 72 hours.

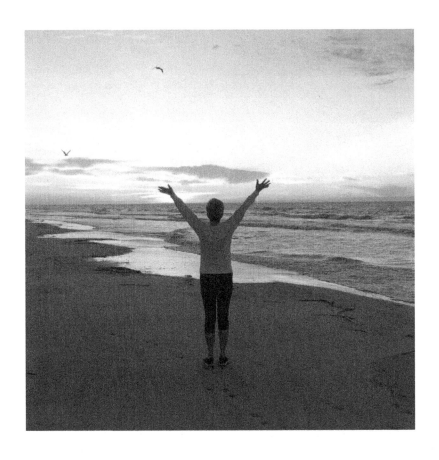

Cleanliness is Next to Godliness

I'm a clean freak. I like things neat and organized. I like to clean. It's always been my thing. I wanted nothing more, however, than a clean PET scan, and that had a lot more to do with my oncologist and the Man upstairs than it had to do with any tasks I could complete. Fortunately, Dr. Chua and God must be clean freaks, too.

I AM CANCER FREE!

One More Perk

Thank you for indulging me as I traveled my journey through six months of sickness. I hope you shared a few laughs along the way.

Visit www.dianabosse.com to order additional books for friends, family members, co-workers, teachers, the mail carrier and your trash collector. Not only will they think you are thoughtful, you'll be doing a good deed as a portion of the proceeds help:

- Research efforts of the Alzheimer's Association (www.alz.org). After all, this is my first passion and the organization that employs me. Plus, I have some pretty outlandish fundraising goals and it would make me look good.

- Cancer research through the Leukemia & Lymphoma Society (www.lls.org). My wish is for as many people as possible to have positive outcomes after a cancer diagnosis.

The rest goes to me. I'm trying to recoup my medical expenses and pay for that Viking River Cruise, remember?

To your health!

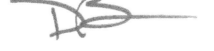

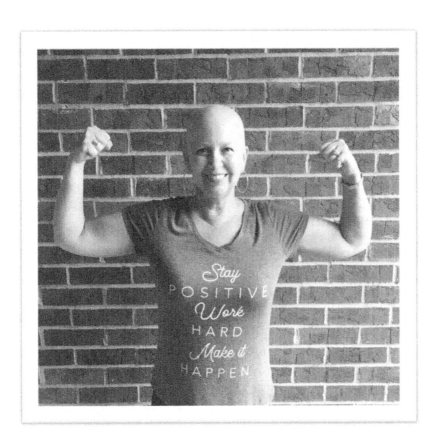

About the Author

Diana Bosse has jotted notes in her diary, written hundreds of grocery lists and published a few articles in company newsletters as well as *The Cincinnati Enquirer, The Island Packet, Ladies Home Journal* and *Women's Day.* This book is a really big deal for her.

Diana grew up on a cul-de-sac in a small Midwestern town in what she refers to as "the last great era to be a child"—the 1960's. She attended grade school and high school where she "didn't learn a thing, but had a great time," then went on to drop out of graphic design school in the early 1980's.

For twenty-five years she worked in the corporate world for the same company where she made a decent living without a college degree and was able to travel to amazing cities such as Atlanta, Dallas, New York, Seattle and Hong Kong on the company dime. Not too shabby for a kid that thought Gatlinburg, Tennessee was the edge of the earth.

Diana currently does meaningful work for an incredible organization—the Alzheimer's Association of Greater Cincinnati.

She lives in Loveland, Ohio with her tolerant husband, Steve, and equally tolerant cat, Madison Grace. All three enjoy spending as many weeks as possible in Maddy's big litter box by the sea, Hilton Head, South Carolina.

This book is the result of someone who once told Diana she was the funniest person she had ever met. Amy obviously needs to expand her social circle. As for Diana, the comment went to her head.

Made in the USA
Monee, IL
15 February 2021